Death, dying, and social differences

Edited by

David Oliviere
Director of Education and Training
St Christopher's Hospice, Sydenham, London, UK

And

Barbara Monroe
Chief Executive
St Christopher's Hospice, Sydenham, London, UK

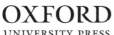

OXFORD
UNIVERSITY PRESS

OXFORD
UNIVERSITY PRESS

Great Clarendon Street, Oxford OX2 6DP

Oxford University Press is a department of the University of Oxford.
It furthers the University's objective of excellence in research, scholarship,
and education by publishing worldwide in

Oxford New York

Auckland Cape Town Dar es Salaam Hong Kong Karachi
Kuala Lumpur Madrid Melbourne Mexico City Nairobi
New Delhi Shanghai Taipei Toronto

With offices in

Argentina Austria Brazil Chile Czech Republic France Greece
Guatemala Hungary Italy Japan South Korea Poland Portugal
Singapore Switzerland Thailand Turkey Ukraine Vietnam

Published in the United States
by Oxford University Press Inc., New York

© Oxford University Press 2004

The moral rights of the author have been asserted

Database right Oxford University Press (maker)

First published 2004
Reprinted 2005 (twice)

A catalogue record for this book is available from the British Library

ISBN 0 19 8527756 (Pbk)

10 9 8 7 6 5 4 3

Typeset by Cepha Imaging Pvt. Ltd., Bangalore, India
Printed in Great Britain
on acid-free paper by
Biddles Ltd., King's Lynn, Norfolk

This book is dedicated to Frances Sheldon, Macmillan Senior Lecturer in Psychosocial Palliative Care, University of Southampton, whose practice, writing, and research has improved the support offered to the dying and those close to them and has informed and inspired the work of so many health and social care professionals.

Foreword

David Clark

In many countries of the world today palliative care is gaining increasing attention as a specialized field of activity within health and social care. There are expanding numbers of services; training and accreditation programmes; a growing research and professional literature; and a plethora of national and international conferences and associations—all bearing witness to hard won achievement and recognition. Yet, despite its claims to consider the 'whole person' and to promote 'multi-professional' care underpinned by 'inter-disciplinary' understanding, few would deny that in palliative care, as in other parts of the health care system, it is often the medical model that predominates, and that opportunities for improving all round care can be lost as a result. With this come the dangers of a lack of attention to 'personhood' and a tendency to see the individual as somehow detached from the social context. There is also the risk that 'patients' and those close to them, however unintentionally, may be reduced to a set of readily categorizable symptoms and pathologies. It is a concern to rectify this imbalance that seems to lie at the heart of this book, and that is what makes it important reading.

During the early 1950s it is possible to detect the first green shoots of a new and concerted professional interest in the care of the dying. A particularly important feature of this was the perspective of social workers and almoners that did much to shape the discussion.[1] On both sides of the Atlantic, important studies demonstrated the problems and difficulties encountered by dying people and those close to them and a picture was revealed of dying and bereavement as profoundly *social* experiences shaped by a variety of factors, including material and cultural circumstances, attitudes to suffering and terminal illness, as well as socially patterned perceptions of the help that might be available. Over time however, as palliative care has consolidated, there is a sense that such perspectives have come to hold less attention in the minds of practitioners. Yet despite the preoccupations

[1] Saunders C (2001) Social work and palliative care—the early history. *British Journal of Social Work*, 31:791–9.

of modern palliative medicine with matters of symptom control and advanced pain management—a vital but necessarily circumscribed set of issues—it is in the main the social dimensions of care in the face of mortal illness that preoccupy most of the people most directly affected. And that is why this book is particularly welcome, providing as it does such a range of contributions to matters of social *difference* at the end of life.

It is a book that encapsulates several important themes and issues. We are offered an exploration of the situation of those sometimes termed 'the disadvantaged dying'—persons locked out of access to the best care at the end of life by virtue of their primary disease, their ethnicity, where they live, or some related form of discrimination, prejudice, or social exclusion. The book pays due attention to the structural forces—class, racism, ageism—that can shape these experiences; but it also reminds us that whilst the dying process can reveal and highlight social difference, death can also be a great leveller: the one experience that we all face and in which the potential for asserting our common humanity is enormous. The book is likewise a testimony to the importance of policy innovation and the power of legislation. Many of its chapters are peppered with references to key reports, the work of expert groups, landmark policy changes, and reforms to service organization and delivery. In that sense it contributes to a longer view of the issues involved in the care of seriously ill and dying people and reminds us that, whilst much remains to be done, a great deal has also been achieved.

David Tasma, the survivor of the Warsaw ghetto who came to die in a post-war London hospital, where he was cared for by Cicely Saunders, was a social and economic migrant, his life shaped by global forces of war and ideology. Since his death in 1948, the social make up of the United Kingdom has been transformed in dramatic ways. Changing patterns of employment and unemployment, population ageing, migration and immigration, ethnic diversity and an altered religious landscape are just a few illustrations. To these can be added the shifting and fractured identities and cultural forces of postmodernity, globalization, and the creation of cyberspace. And of course there are the omnipresent matters of individualism, consumerism, and appeals to autonomy, choice and market relationships. The chapters of this book draw attention to some of these issues, so often overlooked by mainstream palliative care, but which are now beginning to gain notice and which will, perhaps more than anything else, shape the character of palliative care for the next generation of service users and providers.

I am grateful to Barbara Monroe and David Oliviere for giving me the opportunity to say something about this important new collection of writings—one which they have brought together with such imagination and skill. When I received the manuscript of the book, in February 2004, I noticed instantly, and very much appreciated, the dedication to Frances Sheldon. Sadly, just a few weeks later, Frances had died and the world of palliative care had lost one of its greatest advocates for the very people whose problems and experiences are explored in these chapters. The commitment to fairness, equality and human dignity that is echoed in so much of what we read in this book was central to the work of Frances Sheldon, who will be remembered by many as an outstanding leader in the palliative care field. I welcome the arrival of the book just as I mourn the passing of Frances: in a spirit of hope that one day, everyone requiring care at the end of life will find their needs met and their human frailties acknowledged—whatever their social circumstances.

Lancaster, March 2004

Contents

Contributors

Mary Blanche
Head of Service
Asylum Seeker Service Unit, Kent County Council

Maggie Bolger
Head of Business and Administration Training
H M Prison Service

David Clark
Professor of Medical Sociology and Director of the International
    Observatory on End of Life Care
Institute for Health Research, Lancaster University

Katherine Cox
Social Worker
St John's Hospice

Maggie Draper
Social Worker
St Leonard's Hospice

Chris Endersby
Looked After Children Co-ordinator
Kent County Council

Shirley Firth
Hon. Research Fellow
Centre for Ethnic Minority Studies, SOAS, University of London

Donal Gallagher
Social Worker
Wisdom Hospice

Max Henderson
Liaison Psychiatrist and Clinical Research Fellow
St Christopher's Hospice and Institute of Psychiatry and
Maudsley Hospital

Linda McEnhill
Head of Family Support and Chair, Palliative Care and Learning
Disability Network
St Nicholas' Hospice

Ann McMurray
Social Work Manager
Wisdom Hospice

Barbara Monroe
Chief Executive
St Christopher's Hospice

David Oliviere
Director of Education and Training
St Christopher's Hospice

Malcolm Payne
Director of Psychosocial and Spiritual Care and Emeritus Professor
St Christopher's Hospice, Manchester Met University

Sheila Payne
The Palliative and End of Life Care Research Group
University of Sheffield

Chris Wood
Social Worker
St Gemma's Hospice

1

Introduction: working with death, dying, and difference

David Oliviere and Barbara Monroe

Human beings are social animals, embedded within social systems, kinship networks, and cultural groups.

Sheila Payne 2004

Responsiveness to individual need and circumstance and attention to issues of cultural sensitivity is at the heart of palliative care. Government, professionals and individuals express commitment to a vision of appropriate medical care and individualized support being available to all dying people whenever they need it and whoever and wherever they are. The National Health Service report 'Building on the best' (2003) asserts, 'We will train staff to ensure that in time all people at the end of life will be given a choice of where they wish to die and how they wish to be treated.' However, despite the assertions, for much of society 'disadvantaged dying' (Clark and Seymour 1999) is still the norm. 'Death has 100% incidence' (Doyle 1994); no category or class of person is exempt. Yet for many groups, communities and individual patients, the major advances in palliative and end of life care have not touched their lives. The allegation made over a decade ago that palliative care provides 'deluxe dying' for the privileged few (Douglas 1991) remains a challenge for all service providers.

Many sectors of our diverse communities do not have good access to palliative care, or receive services that are at best very patchy (Clark and Seymour 1999). Well-meaning attempts to protect children continue to leave them ignored and isolated as they face bereavement; people with learning disabilities are sometimes denied information; prisoners with advanced illnesses often end their lives in far from adequate medical conditions, minority

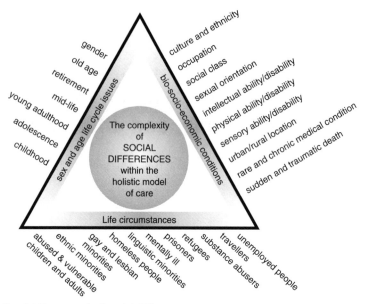

Fig. 1.1 Framework of social differences.

ethnic communities still have unequal access to good care; the needs of refugees and asylum seekers with traumatic past experiences often remain invisible. Add to these examples patients with particular health conditions, such as dementia, psychiatric illness, or non-malignant illness; those who are in a variety of specific social circumstances, for example, those at risk of abuse or who abuse substances; and the different identities based on gender, sexuality, age, class, ability; and a huge multiplicity of need based on social differences is demonstrated. The challenge for palliative care providers and commissioners is not only discerning and responding to the needs and wants of these groups, but also recognizing the variation within the groups themselves.

This book challenges the existing assumptions and models surrounding the delivery of specialist palliative care. It questions the extent to which we are meeting the vision of individualized responsiveness that we espouse. Much of the literature and basic professional assumptions of palliative care are defined by mainstream attitudes about death. Despite our avowed cultural sensitivity, a 'heroic script' (Seale 1995; Walter 1999) defines much of what we do with an insistence on independence, autonomy, and disclosure. How do we provide appropriate care for minority ethnic and religious groups, which are diverse within themselves? What training for professionals will help us to examine our own prejudices and to work appropriately with the conflicts that arise as we work, for example, with groups that favour patriarchal decision-making, or where informed consent for women seems a long way off? What roles should context and relativism properly play in our decision-making? How should we respond to the suggestion that our vaunted cultural sensitivity should give way to a more assertive agenda of race equality (Gunaratnam 1997)?

Physical and psychological characteristics vary widely from person to person. Social and spiritual features shape even more finely the uniqueness of each human being and their preferred mode of dying. Despite almost four decades of the hospice and palliative care movement, and the increasingly widespread acceptance of its messages, the social aspects of end of life care remain little understood and poorly defined (Field 2000; Sheldon 2003). Many writers and researchers comment on the related dimension of 'culture' (Sheldon 1997; Firth 2001) but the strictly social aspect of palliative care is a relatively neglected area. The uniqueness of the 'social person' within the whole person model needs further definition. This uniqueness is informed by the interaction of life circumstances and the differences that society itself constructs. Field, in a National Council briefing paper (2000), 'What do we mean by psychosocial?', challenged the palliative care community to divide the term 'social' from the 'psychological', suggesting that the label 'psychosocial' denied the full range of phenomena that make up social and that the psychological had tended to dominate. Improving the assessment and intervention related to social aspects of patients' and carers' lives involves a paradigm shift in palliative care. Field asserts that, 'for palliative care to be fully effective its practitioners must recognize that for its clients the meaning, experience, and expression of their terminal illness is shaped and influenced by the communities within which they live. The social fabric of their lives is central to how they make sense of their illness experiences, the meanings they draw upon to understand these, and the range of resources they can call upon to help them manage them.' A shift in understanding away from a predominantly individual model to a more structural perception of patients' lives and their social components is overdue. Structural inequality relates to legal, political, and economic considerations. History also shapes health policy and in turn impacts on the resources and quality of service available to dying individuals and their carers.

Our research agendas can further limit the development of appropriate services. For example, research around carers' needs has tended to focus on the practical. Meanwhile Sheila Payne, in a chapter in this book, reminds us that the emotional labour of carers and many carers' needs for independent psychological support have been neglected, as has the supportive emotional reciprocity that exists between many dying individuals and their carers. Established models of grief and bereavement care have disenfranchised some men and many lesbian and gay individuals (Doka 1989; Martin and Doka 2000). People with physical and learning disabilities are defined by many as 'other' in order to create distance, and sometimes as 'less deserving' of treatment (McEnhill 2004). Henderson (2004) suggests that some patients' inability to give positive feedback (for example those with dementia) may make them 'unrewarding' as potential recipients of palliative care. Professionals are not immune to the stereotypes of the majority of the population. Are we offering people equal access to 'our' services or to the ones *they* want and need?

Recent publications have developed some of the rhetoric of a more structural approach. The draft report of the National Institute for Clinical Excellence Guidance on Cancer Services 'Improving supportive and palliative care for adults with cancer' (2003) declares that 'the social impact of cancer is considerable'. It refers to the needs of carers and families and to the importance of user involvement. These statements have yet to be translated into practice realities. How will professionals respond to the often conflicting needs of dying individuals, family, and carers, or to the financial rationing of community-based support? How does palliative care best respond to an increased public expectation of quality and choice? As our communities have become increasingly diverse many minorities feel excluded from mainstream services. As Malcolm Payne (2004) elucidates, even government-backed approaches such as 'social exclusion' can in themselves become discriminatory. Palliative care services need to be aware of their responsibility to promote social cohesion. Action and education is necessary to develop more relevant provision.

Many dying individuals and users of care services have long histories of suffering oppression and injustice in addition to their health or social problems. Practitioners need to find ways to respond to the challenge of working with these groups and their mistrust of healthcare systems as a result of their earlier experiences. We must recognize how the processes of engagement and interaction need to empower before effective care can be delivered. Listening to users' narratives can help us to challenge our own perceptions.

It is important that we now view palliative care within a structural analysis of society, rather than simply as a particular specialism within a range of solely clinical practice issues. There remain huge conquests to make in translating the rhetoric of progress into practical service delivery for all the groups that make up society and in balancing the realities of health economics against the imperative to provide equitable and individualized care.

References

Clark D and Seymour J (1999) *Reflections on Palliative Care*. Open University Press, Buckingham.

Douglas C (1991) For all the saints. *British Medical Journal* 304:579.

Department of Health (2003) *Building on the Best. Choice, Responsiveness and Equity in the NHS*. Department of Health Publications, London.

Doka K (ed.) (1989) *Disenfranchised Grief: Recognising Hidden Sorrow*. Lexington Books, Massachusetts.

Doyle D (1994) Palliative medicine: a UK speciality. *Journal of Palliative Care* 10(1):8–9.

Field D (2000) What do we mean by 'psychosocial'? Briefing No 4 March, National Council for Hospice and Specialist Palliative Care Services, London.

Firth S (2001) Wider horizons. *Care of the Dying in a Multi-cultural Society*. National Council for Hospice and Specialist Palliative Care Services, London.

Gunaratnam Y (1997) Culture is not enough. A critique of multi-culturalism in palliative care. In Field D, Hockey J, and Small N (ed.), *Death, Gender and Ethnicity*. Routledge, London.

Henderson M (2004) Mental health needs. In Oliviere D and Monroe B (ed.), *Death, Dying, and Social Differences*. Oxford University Press, Oxford.

Martin T and Doka K (2000) *Men don't cry... Women do: Transcending Gender Stereotypes of Grief*. Taylor and Francis, Philadelphia.

McEnhill L (2004) Disability. In Oliviere D and Monroe B (ed.), *Death, Dying, and Social Differences*. Oxford University Press, Oxford.

National Institute for Clinical Excellence (2003) *Guidance on Cancer Services. Improving Supportive and Palliative Care for Adults with Cancer*. NICE, Draft, London.

Payne M (2004) Social exclusion, social class and poverty. In Oliviere D and Monroe B (ed.), *Death, Dying, and Social Differences*. Oxford University Press, Oxford.

Payne S (2004) Carers/caregivers. In Oliviere D and Monroe B (ed.), *Death, Dying, and Social Differences*. Oxford University Press, Oxford.

Seale C (1995) Heroic death. *Sociology* 29(4):597–613.

Sheldon F (1997) *Psychosocial palliative care*. Stanley Thornes, Cheltenham.

Sheldon F (2003) Social impact of advanced metastatic cancer. In Lloyd-Williams M (ed.), *Psychosocial Issues in Palliative Care*, Oxford University Press, Oxford.

Walter T (1999) *On bereavement. The Culture of Grief*. Open University Press, Buckingham.

2

Social class, poverty, and social exclusion

Malcolm Payne

Mortality and health inequalities

We all die; no social differences can exclude us from this natural life event. However, social differences can affect the manner and timing of our death and the experience of bereavement. There is good evidence that in areas of deprivation, people in poverty and of lower socio-economic status (social class) suffer more ill-health and die younger than richer people in higher social classes (Wilkinson 1992, 1996; Eames *et al.* 1993; Ben-Schlomo *et al.* 1996).

But while death is certain and class inequalities in health are clear, how inequality comes to affect people's health is uncertain. Blane *et al.* (1998) suggest that three aspects of social inequality may affect health and social care. First, people's behaviour and culture varies with social class and may affect their health or the health care that they receive. There is good evidence that behaviour, such as smoking, dietary preferences, and capacity to use medical services in an informed way, does affect health, and this sometimes also connects with other differences, such as gender and ethnicity (Field *et al.* 1997). Second, psycho-social processes may affect health. For example, people of lower social class may have more stresses in life and less social support, and so may suffer more stress-related illnesses such as coronary heart disease and depression. However, the ways in which such factors actually affect physical health is unclear. Third, generally people in lower social classes are poorer, so may not be able to afford good food, housing and lifestyle, and work in occupations with greater risks of ill-health and accident. There is a greater risk of dying younger than those in higher classes as a result. All these aspects of social inequality may add to and interact with each other creating the overall pattern whereby on average the poorer die younger than the richer.

The lack of clarity about what is happening has led to debate about the impact of poverty and deprivation on health, a debate driven by political ideology in the absence of full understanding. In this political debate, the concept of social exclusion has been deployed by the New Labour government in power in the UK since 1997 as a symbol of its general approach to deprived communities. It has sought to develop neo-liberal policies that focus on raising the general level of economic activity, in particular employment, and social cohesion in deprived communities, in the hope that this will have an impact on broader social inequalities. Health inequalities are not a central plank of the government's approach, therefore. I argue in this chapter that this approach to health inequalities is inadequate, and propose that additional action is required to raise social capital in deprived areas in ways that will directly affect health (and other social inequalities).

Social inequalities in health and health care also extend to palliative and supportive services. People may not receive services that can help them relieve physical, psychological, social, and spiritual pain and discomfort. This may also prevent them from being able to continue with satisfactory social relationships and resolve social difficulties as they die. Their families and the social and community networks around them may then suffer a poor or extended bereavement because of similar inequalities (Bevan 2002). This has long-term consequences, since difficulties in overcoming one difficult life experience is likely to impair the ability to deal with later crises. One of the earliest studies of catastrophic bereavement, Lindemann's (1944) study of the Coconut Grove fire in Boston, found that people with poor experience of crises in their lives coped worse with death in the fire. Consequently, family pressures and difficulties may arise from the cumulative experience of deaths and their impact on the family and its finances and viability.

Health inequalities

Health inequalities played their part in the foundation of the British National Health Service (NHS). Part of the political impetus for a national system free to all at the point of provision was that the poorest groups in society had been excluded from health care. However, it soon became apparent that poor people continued to be disadvantaged, and the Labour government of the 1970s set up a working party in 1977 to study the reasons for this. The Black Report (1980), when it appeared, was suppressed by the then Conservative government, leading to an outcry. A similar fuss attended the publication of a follow-up report, 'The Health Divide' (Whitehead 1987) published as the last act of the discontinued Health Education Authority in 1987. The reasons for the suppression lay partly in the policy prescription of these reports for a total policy approach to health inequality, rather than the mere provision of health care, and a redistribution of resources and activity towards eradicating inequality. The political objection was Conservative opinion that people had to accept personal responsibility for unhealthy lifestyles, that this was downplayed in the reports, and that the costs associated with the recommendations were unrealistic. In response, supporters of the reports argued that there was a long history of under-funding of British health services, and that there was an economic justification of benefit to the community and economy in funding health care more generously. The reports did consider lifestyle problems, but their supporters argued that the Conservative view put too much emphasis on individualism. Conservative individualism encouraged more people to buy health care in the market and to act on their own unhealthy lifestyles. However, supporters of the reports argued that this was likely to be ineffective without committed government support and co-ordination. Inequality could not be tackled without a political focus on eradicating it (Townsend *et al.* 1988).

Health inequalities, then, were central to a clash of political ideologies about health care and proposed actions were symbolic of the attitude of different ideologies to health care policy. Concern about health inequality has continued. The authoritative Acheson Report on 'Inequalities in Health' (Acheson Report 1998) summarized the position in the later 1990s, and the following account draws on this review of the evidence. Death rates in the UK have been falling for more than a hundred years, and in the last part of the twentieth century, death rates for important diseases, such as lung cancer (in men only), coronary heart disease and stroke, also fell markedly. Life expectancy has risen over the past century, but illness and disability have often affected this longer life, since an increasing proportion of people report life-limiting illness. Inequalities measured by death rates, life expectancy, and ill-health were marked and had not decreased. In spite of considerable economic growth in the last half of the twentieth century, and in spite of these improvements in expectation of life the social inequalities in life expectation have at best stayed the same; generally they have worsened. People in the poorest fifth of the population relied more on income support from social security allowances, were more likely to be unemployed, to be lone parents with children, to be disabled or elderly and to live in social housing. Also, Pakistanis and Bangladeshis were more likely to be represented in the poorest fifth, suggesting that social exclusion on 'race' lines may be an important factor.

These findings are significant because mortality from all causes is statistically related to deprived areas and conditions; the poorer the area the worse the mortality (Townsend 1979; Townsend et al. 1988). There is not enough evidence to prove causation and there is evidence that most of the health inequality derives from the concentration of people with adverse personal and household socio-economic factors in their lives (Sloggett and Joshi 1994). Townsend's approach has been criticised on technical grounds (Piachaud 1987). However, ill-health is clearly associated with poverty and social deprivation in particular communities and areas. Moreover, the inequality between areas is worsening. An important study of poor people in the north of England showed between 1981 and 1991 that mortality in the higher social classes improved and mortality in the lower social classes stayed the same or worsened (Phillimore et al. 1994; Townsend et al. 1988). There is evidence that people living on low incomes and state benefits do not have sufficient resources to buy food or to meet other household costs necessary for good health. This is particularly so for children's nutrition and elders' eating, diet, and access to services where there is poor physical mobility.

The effects of poverty in deprived communities on health persist throughout life. In a striking study, Dorling et al. (2000) compared poverty in London based on analysis of Charles Booths' survey in 1896 with the situation at the 1991 Census. Mortality, the rate of death, in diseases related to deprivation was predicted more strongly by the distribution of poverty in 1896 than that in 1991. All cause mortality in people over 65 was slightly more strongly related to the geography of poverty in the nineteenth century than to the 1991 figures.

However, deprived areas are not the only factor in health inequality. In a series of studies of the British civil service, Marmot and his colleagues (Marmot et al. 1984, 1991; Marmot and Shipley 1996) showed health inequalities associated with civil service grade: the lower the grade the worse the health care outcome. These inequalities persisted into retirement and were mirrored by social class measured by car ownership.

The Joseph Rowntree Foundation publishes regular reviews of information about progress on tackling poverty, and maintains a poverty website (http://www.poverty.org.uk/intro/index.htm). Its most recent report at the time of writing (Palmer et al. 2002) shows that Scotland had the highest proportion of premature deaths for men. A third of its local authorities had high mortality rates for men, compared with a tenth in England. While suicide rates are generally dropping, this fall has also not affected Scotland, where suicide rates are three times higher than in England and Wales. Young men (aged 15–24) are four times as likely as young women to commit suicide, and young men with manual backgrounds are twice as likely to commit suicide as those from non-manual backgrounds. The Foundation comments that the government's Public Service Agreement for 2002 does not consider health inequalities, except as part of Health Action Zones. It is not clear whether such a geographically based approach will have effects on health inequalities in the wider population.

To summarize, in the UK there is a long-standing concern and continuing evidence of health inequalities. These inequalities are geographical: some areas of the country face greater health problems and have less health care provision than others. These inequalities are also social: poverty and social exclusion are connected with health inequality. This is directly relevant to death, since poor people die earlier than well-off people. This means that death is likely to have a strong social impact on their lives. People in poor families are more likely to be brought up against death more powerfully and at younger ages as compared with richer families because their family members die sooner and their young men commit suicide or die more often in accidents than well-off people.

The UK reflects international trends (World Bank 2000). In 1960 per capita GDP (a measurement of national wealth) in the 20 richest countries was 18 times that of the poorest 20 countries. By 1995, this figure had increased to 37 times, so inequality between countries continues to grow. Inequality within countries has generally grown since the 1850s, and growth in inequality has continued to the present, but not so steeply as in the 19th century. There is no association between economic growth and reduction of income inequality. Whether inequality reduces as an economy grows depends on complex interactions between social change (such as higher participation by women in an economy), social policy, market changes and legal and institutional changes. All the evidence is that reductions in inequality have to be made to happen by explicit policy actions.

Health inequalities usually disadvantage poor people everywhere, in rich countries and in poor countries: they die earlier and suffer more ill-health than rich people. Wagstaff's (2002) report for the World Health Organisation suggests that there is a cycle of effects: poor people have poor access to health services and knowledge about health, and live in poor conditions. They cannot afford living conditions and nutrition that support good health, and often live in environments that expose them to health risks, do not offer community and family support and have poor access to poor quality health services. They may do manual or factory work where there is a greater risk of injury than office work; they may live in more polluted environments. Consequently, they suffer ill-health and malnutrition, which leads to loss of wages, higher health care costs and greater vulnerability to serious illness. This in turn adds to their poverty and the cycle starts again. Although little is known about how inequalities affect health provision, inequalities in health and in the use of health services reflect inequalities between individual and households such as income, location (e.g. distance from health care facilities), and housing. To combat inequalities, action affecting the supply side (e.g. availability, accessibility, and attractiveness of health care services) and the demand side (e.g. knowledge, awareness, and acceptance of health information) is necessary (Wagstaff 2002). A series of American studies by Kawachi, Kennedy and colleagues (Kennedy *et al.* 1996; Kawachi *et al.* 1997; Lochner *et al.* 2001) show that high mortality is as associated with deprived communities as in Britain, but produce some evidence that this derives from poor social cohesion, with the poor environment of deprived communities forming a social context in which there is an accumulation of individuals with health problems.

Providing universal health services free at the point that a patient receives them is not the complete answer to these problems, contrary to the views of the supporters of the Black Report. World-wide evidence shows that the better-off usually gain more from health care services than the worst off, especially for secondary and tertiary services like hospital and palliative care services. Various ways of targeting services at the poorest present problems. Direct targeting (involving means testing, that is checking the income of applicants for services) and category targeting (providing services to only particular populations many of whom are known to be poor) both present problems. They may miss high proportions of people in need and sometimes raises resistance from those outside the targeted groups (Gwatkin 2003). However, Gwatkin (2003) shows that some countries in Latin America have been successful with policies of careful targeting of free services for poor people within comprehensive health provision. Continual adaptation and development of provision to achieve health objectives for the poor was most effective. This contrasts with the New Labour approach of downplaying emphasis on tackling health inequalities.

Health inequalities, then, are universal, and they affect health and social care provision in the UK just as much as elsewhere. They are measured in the early death and greater ill-health of poor people. At times, and across the world, governments and health professionals have made efforts to respond to health inequalities, but there has been only patchy commitment and little sustained achievement. Yet the evidence is that sustained and careful policy action is required to tackle health inequalities effectively.

Poverty, class, and health inequalities

Health inequalities are closely associated with social class and poverty. So, if we could sweep away poverty, would we reduce health inequalities? This is the British government's approach. It seeks to tackle general social inequalities, on the assumption that this will have an effect on the complex factors deriving from income inequalities.

Poverty is a complex concept, referring to social situations in which people have low incomes and material resources. It may be individuals, families, other social groups, or larger parts of a population that are in poverty. Whether we see poverty in a situation depends on how we see their social relationships. An elderly person or a child may have no income or financial resources, for example, but if they are living as part of a rich family, we may not think of them as 'in poverty'. Because poverty refers to *low* incomes, whether people are in poverty requires a judgement about what is 'low'. It also requires a comparison: what is low depends on what we see as 'high' or 'medium'.

Judgements about responses to poverty have therefore become ideological and political issues. Debates have centred on the extent to which poverty is absolute or comparative and the causes of poverty (Alcock 1997). Someone in poverty in Britain may have a good income compared with someone in sub-Saharan Africa, but we still regard them as poor in comparison with most British people. Among the reasons for this is that the costs of most purchases in Britain are higher, and that British people have higher expectations of what a reasonable life should be. Byrne (1999) identifies two different aspects of income inequality. One is the distribution of income across whole societies. The main point here is that in the thirty-year period from 1945, inequality between the incomes of different groups in British society (and most other European states) was reduced. During the 1980s and '90s, income inequalities increased everywhere, but particularly in Britain. All incomes improved, but higher incomes increased disproportionately. This is the same pattern identified, above in studies of mortality statistics for different social classes. The second aspect of income inequality is the differentiation between different groups within society. Here we can identify particular groups in particular circumstances who are poor. For example, single parents, who are mostly women, are likely to have low incomes and a high demand for expenditure. People from minority ethnic groups are often poorer than the average, and young people are also financially disadvantaged. However, the position of these groups depends on other aspects of social relationships; they may have families or other social structures around them that mean that we would not see them as poor.

These differences in view are mirrored in explanations of poverty and political response to it. As in much of social science, and as in the discussion of social exclusion above, both individuals and the social structure in which they live contribute to poverty; some explanations focus on one more than another. Individualistic (usually regarded as liberal or neo-liberal) explanations emphasise laziness, disorganization, illness, or disability. The assumption behind these is that individual failure or inability to deal with problems or manage their affairs is the main reason for poverty. The idea of the 'cycle of poverty' is one such (discredited) explanation. According to this view, poor families do not educate and bring up their children with the skills necessary for success in society, thus leading to poverty in later generations. There is evidence from studies in the 1970s that most children did not repeat the poverty of their families and communities, and most poor people did not come from deprived backgrounds (Brown and Madge 1982).

Evidence of growing income inequality in rich societies and similarly growing health inequalities has led some, pre-eminently Wilkinson (1996, 1997a, b), to argue that widening inequalities in any particular society leads to breakdowns in social cohesion, which affects health more strongly than absolute poverty. This is an example applied to health care of the argument about whether relative or absolute poverty is more important for policy. There is some evidence for this view, although Wilkinson (1997b) also quotes one study showing contrary findings.

This and the inadequacy of individualistic, neo-liberal analyses of poverty suggest that how the communities came to be poor needs to be the major focus of explanation. Structural explanations focus on how economic and social systems establish patterns of relationships between groups in society that create social divisions. Payne's (2000) analysis proposes that 'social divisions' are universal in all societies. The way it works is that principles of social organization (such as the status of particular jobs) create long-lasting, socially agreed distinctions between categories of people that become part of the culture and division of material resources in the society. As a result, social divisions confer unequal opportunities to desirable resources and therefore life chances and lifestyles. They are rarely or only slowly breached, and produce shared identities according to perceived differences between divisions.

A social divisions analysis claims that health inequalities would always exist and would connect with cultural, social, and behavioural patterns represented in well-understood divisions. These will have material consequences, and the experience of material differences would enhance cultural differences and identify and solidify the social division. Such an analysis shows why the connection between the social and physical is hard to explain, and why inequalities persist in communities and throughout life. In Marmot's studies of civil servants, the inequalities between high grade policy makers and low grade porters and drivers persist because they become part of the cultural and social assumptions of division that affect all social relations.

Social exclusion

Health inequalities may connect with other aspects of social deprivation and inequality through the mechanism of social divisions or similar social processes. In the 1990s, concern about the way in which several aspects of deprivation and equality may come together in particular individuals or communities has led to increased use of the concept of social exclusion. It has become important in policy discourse because it covers a range of dimensions of inequality and disadvantage and poses the question whether they add together to exclude people from civic, social, economic, and interpersonal participation in society (Lund 2002: 8–9). Under the New Labour Blair government, the Prime Minister's office developed a 'Social Exclusion Unit' in 1997 to co-ordinate government action and research on these problems. It moved to the responsibility of the Deputy Prime Minister in 2002. However, none of its work directly dealt with health issues, being mainly concerned with neighbourhood and community issues where severe deprivation affected many aspects of life and young people (SEU 2003). The impact of social exclusion in the UK is in part because of its importance in policy-making in mainland Europe and the European Union.

The debate on social exclusion covers many different points of view and reveals a lack of agreement about what the concept means. Levitas (1998) identifies three discourses or emphases in debate about social exclusion. Redistributionist views emphasize participation as a social, political, cultural, and economic citizen. These views are more idealistic and aim at social cohesion, and are characteristic of the social democratic approach of welfare regimes in mainland Europe. Social integrationist views emphasize participation in paid employment, and this is an important focus of the

UK Social Exclusion Unit. These views are more pragmatic, and aim at economic participation as the basis of other aspects of inclusion: the assumption is that if people are able to work, they will have the money to participate in other aspects of society. This view has had an impact on policy for unemployed young people, rough sleepers, single parents, and disabled people. Moral underclass views focus on difficulties in the behaviour of poor people, such as crime and behaviour likely to lead to ill-health. This view has had an impact on the priority given to managing crime and asylum seekers to improve the quality of life in poor communities.

Social exclusion as a concept may be useful for some purposes, but less useful in others. The advantages of using the concept are that it draws attention to how disadvantageous social conditions cluster together and have social consequences, affecting the same groups in society. People who suffer disadvantages may become outcasts. Their disadvantages all affect each other, so that poverty excludes people from services, makes it more difficult to make social progress through education and, as we have seen, leads to greater ill-health. If they suffer social exclusion in one area, they are likely to suffer it in other areas. Poverty goes hand-in-hand with inequalities due to gender, 'race', disability, and many other factors that lead to discrimination against particular groups in society. On the other hand, the idea of social exclusion emphasizes social consequences rather than the factors in society that lead to the exclusion. So, instead of tackling poverty through better social security provision, or ill-health through better health services, we are led to worry about social integration. It allows us to see discrimination on grounds of gender, 'race', and disability as a social process, thus neutralizing our personal responsibility to avoid discrimination in ourselves and combat it in others. Emphasizing the idea of social exclusion may similarly weaken the responsibility of institutions in our workplaces and leisure time to combat discrimination in their systems and workforces. It can also lead to 'blaming the victim', since there is sometimes a hidden assumption that people could do something about their own exclusion. Also, the idea of social exclusion may lead us to make assumptions that everything about people's lives will display problems. On the contrary, people who have poor general health because of poverty may have supportive family and community relationships, formed in the adversity that they have faced together.

Health inequalities and palliative care

The general pattern of health inequality also extends to palliative care services provided to dying people and their families and to bereavement services.

There is considerable geographical inequality in provision for palliative care. The *Palliative Care Survey 1999* (NCHSPCS 2000) showed 82% more palliative care in-patient beds in the North West and South East Regions than in Trent, 131% more day centre places in Trent than in London, nearly 100% more home care nurses per million of the population in the South West than in Trent. The ratio of doctors' sessions per million of the population in home care was more than 400% greater in London than in the North West. Only 4% of nurses in the North West, Northern and Yorkshire regions worked in home care teams that provided out-of-hours cover, compared with 45% of nurses in London. There are also class inequalities, which suggest that higher social classes can choose where to die and receive palliative care and supportive services, while working classes have little choice and die in acute hospitals. Sims *et al.* (1997), for example, studied all deaths in the Doncaster area in 1995. Social class 1 and 2 with 15% of cancer deaths contributed 24% of the hospice deaths, 14% of the hospital deaths, and 12% of the home deaths. Social class 3 with 24% of cancer deaths contributed 58% of hospice deaths, 9% of hospital deaths, and 35% of home deaths. Social classes 4 and 5 had 61% of the cancer deaths, but contributed only 18% of the hospice deaths, 77% of the hospital deaths, and 53% of the home deaths.

These patterns of inequality are also characteristic of other countries. A statistical study of all American deaths in 1997 showed that bed availability was the factor that most affected the likelihood of dying in acute care hospital, rather than, as 90% of Americans prefer, at home or in a nursing home. Also, non-white and poorly educated people were more likely to die in hospital. Schnoll *et al.* (2002) studied 700 survivors of cancer and showed that adjustment was better where patients were married, and had a high level of education and income. Much of the concern in the USA has focused on non-white groups, where there is considerable evidence of cultural differences, poor outcomes because of lack of social support associated with poorer education and lower socioeconomic status (Bourjolly and Hirschman 2001) and race discrimination (Thomson 2003). However, there were also practical problems of access. Morrison *et al.* (2000), for example, showed that pharmacies in non-white areas of New York did not carry stocks of opioid analgesics because of fears of theft, fears that were unjustified by police data. A Canadian study in Montreal (Daneault and Labadie 1999) sheds light on the extent to which unequal people are treated better to compensate for their inequality. A retrospective study of 307 patients with advanced HIV disease showed that between 1991 and 1997 patients living in extreme poverty were more likely to complain of severe pain and to die in hospital than patients with a similar clinical profile at diagnosis who were financially secure. An Australian study (Chan and Woodruff 1999) of 120 consecutive patients with advanced malignant disease followed up for six months or until death showed that 92% of those unaware of their diagnosis were non-English-speaking. Control of pain and mood disturbance was worse for non-English-speaking patients and of 102 people who died during the study, no non-English-speaking patients died at home.

In summary, there is some patchy evidence that the assumption that health inequalities are universal, and based on universal social divisions holds true for palliative care as for other areas of health care.

Responding to health inequalities

The universality of health inequalities between social divisions and evidence of patchy policy and professional responses to inequality emphasizes the difficulty of intervening to improve the situation. Lister (2000) identifies two fundamental approaches. One, aiming for everyone to have similar opportunities, is to stress social cohesion, to try to promote integration into mainstream services. An example is trying to ensure that disabled people are enabled to work, thus connecting them with work-based social networks and an income from wages. The alternative, for people already disadvantaged to be brought the same advantages of higher social classes, is to stress social justice. The approach recognizes and tries to tackle power imbalances. An example is legislating to require adaptations to buildings to meet the needs of people with mobility problems, or making special social security allowances available. These two approaches are sometimes complementary, both making a contribution. However, pursuing one and avoiding the other may itself be excluding. For example, some disabled people will never be able to work, so restricting state provision to work development will create a category of people whose needs can never be met.

In relation to death and bereavement, the UK government has attempted both approaches. For example, the Department of Health has implemented a policy that dying people should have a choice about where they die, and financial provision follows this. The government guidance on continuing care funding for people in need of health care outside hospitals (Department of Health 2001), for example, specifically makes provision for patient choice at end of life. This is a social cohesion approach because it seeks to allow people to take part in their ordinary social networks. It also makes provision for funding for hospices and for the special rules for the disability living allowance, which speeds up grants for people with a medical prognosis that they have very little lifetime left.

Pierson (2002) identifies five main strategies for tackling social exclusion. First, we should maximize income and welfare rights. Payne (2002), similarly, argues that this is a primary contribution of social work to multiprofessional settings, and (Payne 2001a, b) integral to the basic understanding of social work as a professional activity. Pierson's second strategy is to strengthen social networks of support for excluded people. Third, it is important to build partnerships between agencies working in the same field and with the social groups and individuals that they serve. Consequently, fourth, participation by the people served in decisions that affect them and in the planning, development, and direction of services is a crucial aspect of inclusion. Finally, developing a knowledge of, working within and helping to develop the communities that provide the context of support for excluded people is essential to drawing in excluded groups to mainstream life, in the same way that children with disabilities have been 'mainstreamed' in ordinary rather than special schools.

Health and social care organizations in Britain and more widely, have pursued equal opportunities and anti-discrimination policies to try to reduce the impact of exclusion on particular groups of people, such as those from minority ethnic groups, women, disabled people, and mentally ill people (Tomlinson and Trew 2002). These have several intentions. First, they seek to alter the personnel and policies of health and social care agencies so that they represent better the population that they serve and consistently think of and consider policies that will avoid social exclusion. As a result, agencies should be less likely to exclude people unwittingly, and should try to avoid giving an impression of being likely to exclude minorities, which might discourage minorities from using them. Second, they use techniques in their treatment and organization which empower excluded groups and individuals to compensate for oppression and disadvantage that they have already suffered and advocate for their needs where services have still to develop non-discriminatory practices.

Conclusion: pursuing equity in all we do

The evidence reviewed in this chapter confirms the need to respond to the way individual poverty entwines with social structures creating powerful cultural and social divisions that generate inequalities in health between individuals and communities. Policy approaches have been inconsistent and disputed, both because it is hard to show how ill-health emerges from inequality and because of disagreements in interpretation and analysis of these complex social relationships.

The argument here is that the concept of social exclusion interpreted in a narrow way will lead only to partial engagement with the complex of policy, community, and personal action required to tackle health inequalities. At the policy level, efforts to address health inequalities worldwide have been patchy, but there is evidence that a consistent focus and preparedness to respond to the twists and turns of constant social change does bring improvement. The interaction of personal poverty and community deprivation is unclear, and the need to adapt policy constantly suggests that a multipronged approach to tackling health inequality is required. Both community-level change in deprived communities and effective work with individual circumstances are crucial elements of the armoury.

Palliative and supportive care during dying and bereavement is no less assailed by the problems of health inequalities than any other area of provision, although the evidence of what is happening is sparser than for health care as a whole. It is likely to require a similar consistent and multilevel approach to ensuring that people may receive the right services at this important time in their lives. Palliative care needs to avoid the risk that patterns of social inequality lead to the rich being able to choose where and how to die and receive comfortable provision, while the poor die in acute hospitals or at home less able to draw on support and care focused on dying and bereavement.

References

Acheson Report (1998) *Independent Inquiry into Inequalities in Health* (Chair: Sir Donald Acheson). TSO, London.

Alcock P (1997) *Understanding Poverty* (2nd edn). Palgrave, Basingstoke.

Ben-Schlomo Y, White IR, and Marmot MG (1996) 'Does the variation in the socioeconomic characteristics of an area affect mortality?' *British Medical Journal* 312(7037):1013–14.

Bevan D (2002) 'Poverty and Deprivation'. In Thompson N (ed.) *Loss and Grief: A Guide for Human Services Professionals*, pp. 93–108. Palgrave, Basingstoke.

Black Report (1980) *Working Group on Inequalities in Health*, In Townsend P and Davidson N (ed.)(1988) *Inequalities in Health: The Black Report: The Health Divide*, pp. 29–213. Penguin, Harmondsworth.

Blane D, Bartley M and Davey Smith G (1998) 'Making sense of socio-economic health inequalities'. In Field D and Taylor S (ed.) *Sociological Perspectives on Health, Illness and Health Care*, pp. 79–96. Blackwell, Oxford.

Bourjolly JN and Hirschman KB (2001) 'Similarities in coping strategies but differences in sources of support among African American and white women coping with breast cancer'. *Journal of Psychosocial Oncology* **19**(2):17–38.

Brown M and Madge N (1982) *Despite the Welfare State*, Heinemann, London.

Chan A and Woodruff RK. (1999) 'Comparison of palliative care needs of English- and non-English-speaking patients'. *Journal of Palliative Care* **15**(1):26–30.

Daneault S and Labadie J-F (1999) 'Terminal HIV disease and extreme poverty: a review of 307 home care files'. *Journal of Palliative Care* **15**(1):6–12.

Department of Health (2001) HSC 2001/015 and LAC (2001)18 *Continuing Care: NHS and Local Councils' Responsibilities*. Department of Health, London, http://www.doh.gov.uk/jointunit/015hsc2001.pdf.

Dorling D, Mitchell R, Shaw M, Orford S, and Smith D (2000) 'The ghost of Christmas past: health effects of poverty in London in 1989 and 1991'. *British Medical Journal* **321**(7276):1547–51.

Eames M, Ben-Schlomo Y, and Marmot MG (1993) 'Social deprivation and premature mortality: regional comparisons across England'. *British Medical Journal* **307**:1097–1102.

Field D, Hockey J, and Small N (ed.) (1997) *Death, Gender and Ethnicity*. Routledge, London.

Gwatkin DR (2003) 'Free government health services: are they the best way to reach the poor?' http://poverty.worldbank.org/files/13999_gwatkin0303.pdf.

Kawachi I, Kennedy BP, Lochner K, Protherow-Stith D (1997) 'Social capital, income inequality, and mortality', *American Journal of Public Health* **87**(9): 1491–8.

Kennedy BP, Kawachi I, and Protherow-Stith D (1996) 'Income distribution and mortality: cross-sectional ecological study of the Robin Hood index in the United States'. *British Medical Journal* **312**:1004–5 (Important correction: 1191).

Levitas R (1998) *The Inclusive Society: Social Exclusion and New Labour*. Macmillan, Basingstoke.

Lindemann E (1944) 'Symptomatology and management of acute grief'. In Parad HJ (ed.)(1965) *Crisis Intervention: Selected Readings*. Family Service Association of America, New York.

Lister R (2000) 'Strategies for social inclusion: promoting social cohesion or social justice?' In Askonas P and Stewart A (ed.) *Social Inclusion: Possibilities and Tensions*. Macmillan, Basingstoke.

Lochner K, Pamuk E, Makuc D, Kennedy BP, and Kawachi I (2001) 'State-level income inequality and individual mortality risk: a prospective, multilevel study'. *American Journal of Public Health* **91**(3):385–91.

Lund B (2002) *Understanding State Welfare: Social Justice or Social Exclusion?* Sage, London.

Marmot MG, Shipley MJ, and Rose G (1984) 'Inequalities in death – specific explanations of a general pattern' *Lancet* i:1003–6.

Marmot MG, Davey Smith G, Stansfeld S, Patel C, North F, Head I, *et al.* (1991) 'Health inequalities among British civil servants: the Whitehall II study' *Lancet* 337:1387–93.

Marmot MG and Shipley MJ (1996) 'Do socioeconomic differences in mortality persist after retirement? 25 year follow up of civil servants from the first Whitehall study', *British Medical Journal* 313(7066):1177–80.

Morrison RS, Wallenstein S, Natale DK, Senzel RS, and Huang LL (2000) '"We don't carry that" – failure of pharmacies in predominantly nonwhite neighborhoods to stock opioid analgesics' *New England Journal of Medicine*, 342:1023–6.

NCHSPCS (2000) *The Palliative Care Survey 1999*. National Council for Hospice and Specialist Palliative Care Services, London.

Palmer G, Rahman M, and Kenway P (2002) *Monitoring Poverty and Social Exclusion 2002*. Joseph Rowntree Foundation, York.

Payne G (2000) 'Social divisions and social cohesion'. In Payne G (ed.) *Social Divisions*, pp. 242–53. Macmillan, Basingstoke.

Payne M (2001*a*) 'Det sociales arbejdes identiter under forandring'. *Tidskrift for Social Forskning* 2(3):4–18.

Payne M (2001*b*) 'Balancing the equation' *Professional Social Work*, January 2002, 12–13.

Payne M (2002) 'Coordination and teamwork'. In Adams R, Dominelli L, and Payne M (ed.) *Critical Practice in Social Work*, pp. 252–60. Palgrave, Basingstoke.

Phillimore P, Beattie A, and Townsend P (1994) 'Widening inequality of health in northern England, 1981–1991'. *British Medical Journal* 308(6937):1125–8.

Piachuad D (1987) 'Problems in the definition and measurement of poverty'. *Journal of Social Policy* 16(2):144–64.

Pierson J. (2002) *Tackling Social Exclusion*. Routledge, London.

Schnoll RA, Knowles JC, and Harlow L (2002) 'Correlates of adjustment among cancer survivors'. *Journal of Psychosocial Oncology* 20(1):37–59.

Social Exclusion Unit (2003) *SEU's work*. http://www.socialexclusionunit.gov.uk/SEUs_work.htm (accessed 2nd August 2003).

Sims A, Radford J, Doran K, and Page H. (1997) 'Social class variations in place of cancer death'. *Palliative Medicine* 11:369–73.

Sloggett A and Joshi H (1994) 'Higher mortality in deprived areas: community or personal disadvantage?' *British Medical Journal* 309(6967):1470–4.

Thomson GF (2003) 'Discrimination in health care', *Annals of Internal Medicine* 126(11):910–12.

Tomlinson DR and Trew W. (2002) *Equalising Opportunities, Minimising Oppression: A Critical Review of Anti-Discrimination Policies in Health and Social Welfare*. Routledge, London.

Townsend P (1979) *Poverty in the United Kingdom: A survey of Household Resources and Living Standards*. Allen Lane, London.

Townsend P, Davidson N, and Whitehead M (1988) 'Introduction to *Inequalities in health*'. In Townsend P and Davidson N (ed.)(1988) *Inequalities in Health: The Black Report: The Health Divide*, pp. 1–28. Penguin, Harmondsworth.

Townsend P, Phillimore P, and Beattie A (1988) *Health and Deprivation: Inequality and the North*. Routledge, London.

Wagstaff A (2002) 'Poverty and health sector inequalities'. *Bulletin of the World Health Organisation* **80**(2):97–105, http://www.who.int/docstore/bulletin/pdf/ 2002/bul-2-E-2002/80(2)97–105.pdf

Whitehead M (1987) The health divide. In Townsend P and Davidson N (ed.) (1988) *Inequalities in Health: The Black Report: The Health Divide*, pp. 215–81. Penguin, Harmondsworth.

Wilkinson RG (1992) 'Income distribution and life expectancy'. *British Medical Journal* **304**:165–8.

Wilkinson R (1996) *Unhealthy Societies: The Afflictions of Inequality*. Routledge, London.

Wilkinson R (1997a) 'Socioeconomic determinants of health: health inequalities: relative or absolute material standards'. *British Medical Journal* **314**(7080):591–5.

Wilkinson R (1997b) 'Comment: Income, inequality and social cohesion'. *American Journal of Public Health* **87**(9):1504–6.

World Bank (2000) *World Development Report, 2000–2001: Attacking Poverty*, Oxfords University Press/World Bank, New York, http://www.worldbank.org/ poverty/wdrpoverty/index.htm

3

Minority ethnic communities and religious groups

Shirley Firth

Death with dignity is a fundamental human right, and in multi-ethnic and religiously diverse Britain, high quality care should be available for all (Gatrad *et al.* 2003). Minority groups know the kind of care they want, and models of a good death, which they want to experience congruent with their religious beliefs and practices. However, the evidence suggests that the numbers receiving hospice and specialist palliative care services fall well below their proportion in the population.

This chapter focuses chiefly on the South Asian and African/African Caribbean communities, as these are the biggest minorities and there is little other research available. It attempts to address concerns about appropriate care, raise issues, points of principle and practice, and offers suggestions for an anti-discriminatory framework for professionals and evolving services.

Culture, ethnicity, and race

The use of words like 'race', 'ethnicity', and 'culture' has been bedevilled by changes in attitudes to their use in different cultural and religious contexts (Gunaratnam 2003). In UK law, 'ethnicity' relates to those with 'a long shared history and a distinct culture ... a common geographic origin or descent from a small number of ancestors; a common language, a common literature; a common religion and being a minority within a larger community' (CEEHD 2003). This definition implies that the majority is not 'ethnic'. Ethnicity is something *they* possess, not *us*. Hence Gunaratnam prefers 'minoritized people' to 'ethnic minorities', with its connotations of 'Otherness'. Many writers prefer the term 'ethnicity' to 'culture' when examining patterns of health and disease as it implies shared biological characteristics. Culture has been blamed for illness and poverty, which can be solved by providing the right education (Pfeffer and Moynihan 1996).

Culture is 'a constellation of shared meanings, values, rituals, and modes of interrelating with others that determines how people view and make sense of the world' (Krakauer *et al.* 2002:204). It includes shared history, religion, food, life-style, and arts. It is dynamic, located in the context of socio-economic conditions. Chattoo *et al.* found palliative care writings assume that culture is 'a fixed and innate attribute to the exclusion of agency and choice; in contrast the white majority community is constructed in terms of the individual, autonomy, and choice, with no discussion of culture' 2002:46). Jones comments, 'The rights of families to medical knowledge and their roles in decision-making are just as valid, inalienable, and crucial to the cultural belief systems of many ethnic minority communities as patient autonomy models are to Western patients' (2003:11). Checklists and fact files tend to ignore aspects of culture other than religion, reify it and reinforce stereotypes (Jones 2003). Chattoo *et al.*'s comparative study showed that many experiences of patients and families were similar from all ethnic groups, and that each individual's experience had to be placed into his/her own context while highlighting areas in which 'ethnic, religious or racial identity [was] significant in making sense' (2002:46).

Who are the minority ethnic people?

In England the minority ethnic population is about 9% of the total (Census 2001). Many were born in the UK. The migration history of each immigrant is different, whether professional, refugee, factory, or public service worker. East African Asians came as families. Bangladeshis, Pakistanis, and Sikhs came to work in manufacturing. When factories closed many Bangladeshis moved to London's East End, where they form one of the most impoverished communities in the UK (Gardner 2002).

West Indians arrived from the 1950s to work in factories, transport, and nursing. Many elders now experience loneliness, isolation, and poverty (Blakemore 2000). Refugees have come from war-torn Europe, Vietnam, Bosnia, Kosovo, Somalia, Congo, Afghanistan, and Iraq. Many have endured torture, physical, emotional, and sexual abuse, facing uncertain futures in an unexpectedly hostile environment. This may prevent them seeking medical help, especially if it hampers claims for asylum, housing and benefits.

Within each 'group' there are immense variations of culture, religion, language, socio-economic status, and education; hence there is no such thing as South Asian, African, Chinese, or Caribbean culture. Most will have experienced racism, prejudice, and stereotyping, whether at personal or institutional levels, as well as multiple changes, losses, and trauma. These factors play a part in attitudes and responses to illness and death.

Family structures

Many cultures are collectivist, the individual less important than caste, tribe, or family. Tse notes, 'The concept of self is a relational one in Chinese culture, and family relations emphasize harmonious interdependence.' (2003:339). Kinship groups provide material, emotional, and spiritual support during life-cycle events; however, they may not provide equal support and care during illness, especially if it is stigmatizing (Chattoo *et al.* 2002).

For many South Asians decision-making is patriarchal. Male power roles are reinforced if the women do not speak English and are dependent upon their husbands or sons to translate. This creates problems for nursing staff who wish to communicate directly with female patients to discuss, e.g. pain relief, while the husbands expect communication to be addressed to them (Gardner 2002). There are real dilemmas between wishing to respect autonomy and informed consent for women, and respecting their situation in their particular context.

Chattoo *et al.* found that despite differences of ideal, norms about caring and family obligations between white and South Asian families, 'caring follows similar processes of negotiation and hierarchy of relationships within close, extended family across ethnic groups' (2002:31), with a similar desire to 'care for our own'. However, joint families are fragmenting, with education increasing social and economic mobility. This affects family life and structures as familiar patterns of responsibility and authority shift.

Health beliefs and explanatory systems

Explanatory systems and health beliefs influence ethnic health patterns, behaviour, and service utilization (Pfeffer and Moynihan 1996). Beliefs about cancer can hinder prevention, diagnosis, and appropriate treatment. Chattoo *et al.* found it was 'largely defined as the unspeakable disease by a majority of both the South Asian and White patients' associated with a slow, painful death (2002:12). Cancer may be associated with death, punishment, evil forces, and contagion, affecting rates of diagnosis. Pakistani Muslims attribute different causes to illness, from the incorrect balance of the bodily elements to the evil eye (*nazar*), *jinns* and magic, but 'ultimately religious beliefs provide the 'final cause' explanation of illness' (Shaw 2000:150). Belief in God's will is not an abdication of individual responsibility for health-seeking behaviour.

It is important to engage with the patients and relatives to understand their perspective, and explain one's own. There may be unrealistic expectations of Western medicine—that medication and going to hospital 'make you better' (Firth 1997). Medicines may be 'seen as being time-limited... so ongoing drugs used in symptom control need further explanation' (Lund 2002:10; see Boyle 1998).

Attitudes to purity are deeply imbedded in many religions. The requirement to be pure for prayer and rituals goes far beyond mere cleanliness, but reflects an attitude of the spirit to align itself with God. The stigma of cancer may be increased by conditions affecting bodily emissions, such as a fungating wound or colostomy, which can have 'further, social and spiritual implications for the notion of a 'whole body' that participates in ritual and religious domains... [which] could result in greater degrees of social isolation due to stigma associated with a leaky or 'unbounded body.' (Chattoo *et al.* 2002:18). The effects of cancer, such as hair and breast loss can thus result in 'a spoiled identity'.

Attitudes to death

While the idea of a 'good death' is quite contentious in western literature, it is a feature of many religions, including the historical Christian *Ars Moriendi* (the art of dying). It is related to choice and control over the time, manner, and place of death (Firth 1997), and to one's spiritual state, relationship to God or Ultimate Reality. It may include offering and receiving forgiveness from God and man, and becoming detached from this life. Because it is important to be conscious, with an unclouded mind, to focus on God or Ultimate Reality, pain-relieving medication may be refused. Death may be anticipated to the day. Good deaths provide cognitive and emotional meaning, enabling both the dying and their relatives to make sense of suffering and death, with an assurance of continuity.

For most South Asians, a good death is located in the sacred space of home, whereas a hospital is a profane place, 'where you go to get better' (Firth 1997). At home it is possible to say goodbye, offer prayers and readings and chant or sing hymns. For a Bangladeshi woman, '...dying at home means that the ... (Quranic Surahs) can be read for you. If *Kolima Shadat* falls on their ears then the dying will remember Allah... people say: 'Allah, when I die let it be with the *Kolimas* in my ears.' (Gardner 2002:195).

An elderly Punjabi woman asked her grandson, 'Make a bed for me on the floor and give me a diva (light) in my hand. I want to go to God' (Firth 1997:58). Good deaths are celebrated, and their narratives become part of the transmission of faith through the family and community, giving the bereaved some idea of the 'place' of the dead. In many cultures the dead live in a parallel world, affecting the living.

Being present at the death, and hearing last words is important in all cultures. The final moments have a profoundly spiritual as well as emotional aspect. Relatives who are told that the dying person is all right and sent home are often devastated to find they have died in their absence (Firth 1997; Gardner 2002).

Rituals have several functions. They connect the participants to God or Ultimate Reality. They may guarantee a place in the next world for the deceased. Hindus who are not able to perform basic rituals like giving Ganges water to a dying patient may subsequently be desperately anxious that the unquiet ghost will cause problems (Firth 1997). From a social perspective, rituals provide cohesion and solidarity for a newly fragmented group. They also enable the dying and living to disengage from each other, and give shape to grief and mourning.

Many immigrants wish to return 'home' to die or be buried. Bangladeshi kin at home want to see the body and visit the grave, but there are also issues of identity (Gardner 2002), reflecting feeling alien and uprooted in the new country, outweighing the tradition that one should be buried where one has died. This is changing with the establishment of Muslim burial grounds in Britain. Hindus and Sikhs may have ashes taken to the Ganges, but some Hindus have created their own sacred space in British rivers (Firth 1997).

Many groups, including Africans, feel that hospital is a better place to die than home, because it provides hope. For many Chinese, death at home creates bad luck and pollution (Boyle 1998). Johnson *et al.* (2001) found preferences about where to die were not linked with ethnicity or culture, but based on personal choice. No one should die alone. It is essential to ascertain what *individuals* feel is appropriate for them, rather than assume that members of a particular 'culture' want the same thing.

Access

Many studies suggest that minority ethnic access to palliative care services is lower than their proportion in the local community would suggest (Firth 2001). Reasons include ignorance about services, lack of accessible and appropriate information, and little confidence in the ability of services to understand or meet their needs. They may perceive hospices as places where white people die, be anxious about appropriate religious and cultural care, and concerned about communication. Referrals can be seen as a death sentence for the patient, stigmatizing, with loss of honour for families who allow their relative to go to a hospice. In areas with small numbers of minority ethnic groups provision may be thought unnecessary (Webb *et al.* 2000). Other barriers include experience of racism from staff and other patients, insensitivity and lack of cultural awareness.

Many GPs and hospital consultants are not referring patients to palliative care services, often because they believe the families would 'care for their own' (Karim *et al.* 2000). Since the language of the patient is not on referral forms this creates further difficulties. Asian or other minority ethnic doctors referring fewer patients to palliative care, may be ignorant of services (Choudhury 1999). Minority ethnic doctors, often Western-trained, are no more homogeneous as a group than the communities they serve, and they may be making unjustifiable assumptions about patients from different or lower caste backgrounds. There may also be fewer resources and staff for single-handed inner-city GPs (Gerrish 1999).

Lower access rates may reflect lower rates of most types of cancer among most minority ethnic groups, the rates later converge with those of white people. (Harding and Rosato 1999). However, Irish people, an 'invisible minority' have the second highest cancer rates in England and Wales, after the Scots, twice the rate of prostate cancer, and high rates of leukaemia (Tilki 1998).

Coronary heart disease, diabetes, and hypertension, which cause most concern for minority ethnic patients are not yet considered for specialist palliative care services, raising questions about need and equity (Choudhury 1999).

For African HIV/ AIDS sufferers, stigma is a further barrier to access. They present later for medical consultations than the white population, because of '…the fear of being experimented upon, lack of confidence in drugs tested only on Caucasians, distrust of the medical profession, and fears of discrimination (Erwin and Peters 1999:1519). The lack of accurate data presents a challenge to palliative care services (Aspinall 2000), and further research is needed into appropriate provision for HIV/AIDS patients from minority ethnic groups throughout the country.

Carers

Caring for dying relatives at home is a matter of honour and integrity for many families; failure or inability to do so creates stigma and loss of face.

It is a sacred duty with profound religious implications and 'implications for moral identity ... of fulfilling certain obligations ... set into the context of the respect of the wider community' (Chattoo *et al.* 2002:30).

Because of changes in the extended family system, home care may be impossible. Chattoo *et al.* found those without an extended family 'felt particularly isolated and vulnerable ... Lack of access to English as an important cultural resource, old age, illness-related impairment, and immobility could further accentuate their sense of isolation and vulnerability in facing a serious condition' (2002:20).

South Asian men tend to be the decision-makers; in practice wives and daughters-in-law, often with little English, usually undertake the physical tasks (Spruyt 1999; Lund 2002). Tensions can arise when an elder needs care from a female relative with quite different expectations, especially if she has children born in Britain. In cross-cultural marriages, there may also be different expectations of care for the sick and elderly. Multi-generational Pakistani and Bangladeshi families may be in situations with high unemployment and poverty, and many young children (Blakemore 2000). Spruyt (1999) found the caring role of many Bangladeshi children had a negative impact, especially if they had to give up school or work.

Carers need information about what is going on and what is available, support with language, advocacy and finance, practical help and emotional support (Johnson *et al.* 2001). Financial help is sometimes needed both for dying individuals and bodies to be returned 'home'.

Disclosure and truthtelling

In palliative care, professionals may have moral dilemmas over issues of truth telling and disclosure. Chattoo *et al.* observe that the literature

> invokes a prescriptive culture of dying in terms of open awareness and a 'new regime of truth' ... with fixed scripts for the patient and the family for 'coping' and mourning. Any deviations ... are ... 'denial', while some are perceived as being 'at risk' for mourning (2002: 16.)

In 'familial' cultures, relatives may expect to make decisions on patient's behalf, usually to maintain quality of life. Protecting the patient from the truth to maintain hope overrides considerations of patient autonomy and the right to know, in keeping with their understanding of the principles of beneficence, non-maleficence, fidelity, respect, and justice (Werth *et al.* 2002). Gardner (2002) suggests this is not just paternalism but, for Bengalis, 'deeply held beliefs surrounding individual choice and 'rights' [and]...

concerning the primacy of the family, gender relations, and Bengali ideas of appropriate treatment for the dying' (2001:242). For Hindus there is often a dilemma between needing to know in order to prepare for a 'good death', and non-disclosure 'in case they give up hope', sometimes reflecting the relatives' ambivalence. Johnson *et al.* found South Asians agreeing ' ... that knowledge was better, so that the individual could make his or her preparation, 'make a will', 'get religious', and the family could offer them a good time and make them 'as happy as possible' during their last days, weeks, or months' (2002: 28).

Some Chinese fear that speaking about death will bring it about (Boyle 1998). Staff may be asked to withhold information from the patient. However, patients often know more than their relatives would wish; there may be control issues (Ng *et al.* 2000). The ethics of disclosure is an issue in Judaism. Maintenance of life is a primary mandate, and disclosure could cause patients to lose hope and thus die sooner than they might have done (Katz 2000). The dilemma is exacerbated when there is a question of withdrawing hydration or arranging hospice care, as these involve disclosure, and could hasten death.

Werth *et al.* (2002) stress the importance of professionals explaining their own cultural value system regarding truth-telling and informed consent. They must be willing to negotiate, while being sensitive to verbal and non-verbal cues as to the preparedness of the patients and relatives to discuss things openly.

Communication

Poor communication is cited frequently as a problem by both patients and providers (Johnson *et al.* 2001; Chattoo *et al.* 2002; Randhawa *et al.* 2003). Koffman and Higginson noted that 'Many black Caribbean respondents reported ... that they felt invisible in important decision making' (2001:344). Reliance on relatives to translate, disadvantages both the doctor and the patient. The interpreter may filter, abbreviate, or omit information and tell the doctor or the patient what s/he thinks the other needs to know. Many interpreters are inexperienced with cancer and with giving bad news, and unable to explain health beliefs, medical jargon, body language, and gestures. The use of children is totally inappropriate, disempowering women who depend on them, and unfair on the children (Bowes and Domakos 1995). Using friends or local untrained lay interpreters creates problems of confidentiality and fear of gossip.

Communication also involves body language, cultural rules about courtesy, eye contact, and appropriate behaviour in unequal gender and power relationships. English-speakers with different accents may be judged to be less intelligent (Gerrish *et al.* 1996). Good communication involves patient listening and explaining the diagnosis, prognosis and treatment, to ensure everything is understood (Werth *et al.* see box). Patients may feel powerless and vulnerable, partly because their condition creates pain and fear, but also because of staff attitudes. They have to learn appropriate roles in a social process involving rules, values, and different cultural expectations. Medical staff are equally products of their culture and not just rational, impartial or,

> 'affectively neutral' actors in relationships with patients, while the patients themselves are ... the ones bringing to the encounter emotion, pain, values, and particular cultural attitudes—whether they are English, Welsh, Cypriot or Sikh (Blakemore and Boneham1994:105).

Guidelines for Communication

- ◆ Assess the language that the patient/family use in discussing the illness and disease, including the extent of openness with regard to the diagnosis, prognosis, and death.
- ◆ Determine the locus of decision making. Is it the individual patient, the family or another social unit?
- ◆ Solicit the patient's and family's views about the appropriate location and timing of death, including the preferred role of family members and health care providers.
- ◆ Assess the degree of fatalism or activism within the patient and family. Is there acceptance regarding future events or a desire to control aspects of these events?
- ◆ Consider gender issues and power relationships within the decision-making unit.
- ◆ Assess religious beliefs of the patient and family, focusing on the meaning of death, the existence of an afterlife, and belief in miracles. Also establish beliefs about the body after death (e.g. who owns the body and how is it to be treated?).
- ◆ Assess how hope is maintained within the family and negotiated with health care providers. What are the cultural meanings associated with maintaining hope?

Werth *et al.* 2002:214

Interpreters, bilingual support workers, and patient advocates

The question of adequate interpreting and advocacy schemes recurs again and again in the literature (Firth 2001). Interpreters have to be bicultural *and* bilingual (Somerville 2001), so that they understand the ways both patients and professionals think. South Asians want more interpreters and advocates with a 'mutual understanding of religion and culture; the ability of a professional to appreciate and 'read' a whole way of life" (Randhawa *et al.* 2003:27).

Somerville (2001) argues that the use of interpreters masks the need for bilingual staff and blocks the drive to recruit and train them. However, ethnic minority staff should not become interpreters at the cost of their other work (Firth 1997). Nor should it be assumed that they can 'speak for' their culture. Differences in education, culture, and class may be as significant as the language.

Properly trained, employed advocates go some way to meet these needs. The Health Advocacy for Minority Ethnic Londoners Project found piecemeal and disconnected services. This is also true nationally. The priorities identified were to fund a health advocacy network, develop agreed standards for the delivery of health advocacy services, explore ways of improving the funding base for health advocacy services, and provide support for the development of accredited training (Silvera and Kapasi 2000).

Barriers to recruitment are low pay, low status, the lack of professional recognition, or of a proper career structure. One South Asian advocate and outreach worker, with multiple roles, receives less pay than the gardener at the hospice where she works. Most advocacy courses in Britain do not specialize in palliative care. However, the Capacity Project, at the University Hospital Birmingham NHS Trust, is designed to help people with cancer access services. A team of community advocates from seven communities, are trained in cancer and palliative care issues, supporting people at any stage of cancer, with feedback to service providers. Funded by the New Opportunities Fund, advocates help people understand and explore the options available to them, explain treatment and procedures, and address difficulties of access (Mike Wright, personal communication 2003).

Spiritual and religious support

Religious and spiritual support are part of the fundamental philosophy of palliative care. Research suggests that adequate spiritual support for dying patients plays a large part in alleviating distress around death

(Chibnall *et al.* 2002). While patients prefer to be ministered to by their own co-religionists, they are not always available. A religious faith does not mean that someone will not have spiritual needs, doubts and questions (Firth 2001), which can be helped by culturally skilled and empathetic care. However chaplaincy provision is inadequate. The low levels of funding and numbers of volunteer chaplains 'suggest that spiritual care is largely operationalized within a Christian context and tradition. The absence of any assessment of the patient's spiritual, religious, and cultural requirements in 29% of hospitals, and the lack of multifaith guidelines in 40% of hospitals add weight to this point' (Wright 2001:240). Christian chaplains, especially Anglicans, assume the role of spiritual broker for all faiths 'who by virtue of establishment 'hold on to' everyone's 'spiritual bit' [which] does raise questions about the role of others ... brokerage has a subtle impact on the development of *formal* mechanisms for including others in the team. It diminishes an awareness of the need for religious leaders from other traditions, as the broker oversees meeting the needs of all' (Orchard 2001:152).

There are no traditional equivalents to the pastoral role in other faiths. Lie (2001) suggests new models should evolve, seeking 'other creative possibilities—the social worker, link worker, counsellor, teacher, community specialist, health care professional—each with a deeply held religious faith and practice' (Lie 2001:188). Rabbis now add pastoral care to their teaching role (Gilliat-Ray 2001) and the Muslim Council is providing NHS funded training for Muslim chaplains, paid for by the NHS.

Johnson *et al.*'s (2001) informants insist that while the communities themselves should help their own patients and families, the National Health Service should provide this, with religious leaders brought into existing multidisciplinary teams. Birmingham Hospital Trust has had Muslim men and women chaplains since the 1990s, with more limited funding for Hindu, Sikh and Jewish advisors. The North London Hospice was founded as a multifaith hospice, with three Christian chaplains, a Jewish and a Muslim chaplain. A Hindu Chaplain sees Hindu patients when needed, covering for other Chaplains as necessary. A Spiritual and Cultural Services Facilitator has recently been appointed to support the chaplaincy, ensuring relations with faith groups are maintained, and also to liaise with other ethnic and cultural groups, providing feedback to the hospice about specific cultural and ethnic needs.

Outreach and information

Doctors and primary care teams, as gatekeepers, may fail to inform patients and families of palliative care provision because it is deemed inappropriate

(Karim *et al.* 2000; Koffman and Higginson 2001). Randhawa *et al.* found that patients obtained information on an ad hoc basis from surgeries, Macmillan nurses, other professionals, through posters and leaflets, and 'learned very little through face-to-face interaction' (2003:27). They knew little of translated material, or audio or video cassettes in their own languages. Television, radio, the internet, and videos are valuable ways of disseminating information, particularly for people who are not literate.

This approach has been made in Birmingham by the South Asian Palliative Care Awareness Arts Project, SAPCAA, with live drama and a video, *Humara Safar*, 'Our Journey', the story of a South Asian elder with cancer, who is reluctant to accept palliative care services. Although in Hindi, it has been used with a wide range of South Asian groups in the West Midlands. The Bollywood type title has attracted large audiences. The project, funded by the New Opportunities Fund, consulted communities as to what they wanted and needed, and provides a mixture of light relief and health education about cancer and palliative care.

Despite reservations about hospices, many minority ethnic people have responded positively to outreach programmes and good information. When they visit hospices or experience them first hand, they are impressed with the care offered, especially the possibility of respite care (Karim *et al.* 2001; Simmonds *et al.* 2001). Where outreach workers and advocates are already in place, such as Compton Hospice (Wolverhampton) and Acorns Children's Hospice (Birmingham), they liaise with local communities, and the minority ethnic intake at Acorns is commensurate with the proportion of local community. Rotherham Hospice has a Multicultural Link Palliative Care Nurse with the tasks of research into minority ethnic needs, participating in hospice at home, improving access, and providing educational programmes for staff and minority ethnic groups.

Cultural competence and cultural safety

The concepts of cultural competence and cultural safety were developed by Leinger and Ramsden (Coup 1996), respectively, to move beyond practical skills to attitudinal change. They denote skills and knowledge, which transcend language, ethnicity, culture, and upbringing. They insist also on empowering ethnic minorities themselves to be involved in the development of culturally safe practice in partnership with the majority community (Coup 1996).

Training in cultural competence and safety cannot be left to the half-day session often provided; it needs to be part of mainstream professional education (Gerrish *et al.* 1996), including insights from anthropology and cultural psychology. It requires the development of self-awareness, so that professionals can reflect and examine their own beliefs, responses, and views. It has to include issues of racism and discrimination. This involves 'emotional labour', taking informed risks, trusting to intuition, and self monitoring, and welcoming feedback from colleagues, carers, and patients. By 'referential grounding', professionals are able to see another person as a similar human being to themselves (Gunaratnam *et al.* 1998). This requires actual encounters with local communities *outside* the professional relationship, in the context in which they live and work (Lie 2001).

Empowerment

Many patients and families feel that they have no choices over where to die, or how to care for the dying (Firth 1997). Being unable to communicate, experiences of racism, and not understanding issues around prognosis and treatment, all contribute to feeling helpless and marginalized. If the importance of the family in making end-of-life decisions is discounted, then they will not be able to provide adequate support. It is necessary to be sensitive to varying expectations among patients, practitioners and families to enable them to work together to provide appropriate information and care (Jones 2003).

Empowerment involves engaging with communities to find out what they want and need, and ensuring proper representation at all levels. Commitment and adequate funding are required to employ minority ethnic staff, liaison or outreach workers, and train community advocates or linkworkers with a proper salary and career structure. If, indeed, most minority ethnic patients do want to die at home, this presents a challenge to develop hospice at home programmes.

Conclusion

Even with limited research, there is enough knowledge about minority ethnic needs to establish equitable policies in management, practice, education, and training. This demands commitment of time and money from the top down. Minority ethnic people are not just 'Others' to be accommodated until they learn our ways, but a part of society with as much to offer as to receive. 'The usefulness of the evidence to research, policy and service-user circles contributes to the larger society's dialogue on death and dying more generally, encouraging participation... through consideration of individual and group differences' (Jones 2003). In addition to policies commited to equitable care, nursing and medical education and training should include cultural competence and knowledge, and anti-discrimination as mainstream. Further research into little known groups is needed. The welcome new research projects into Chinese perspectives on Cancer by Sheffield University and Macmillan will throw light on their needs (National Council 2003).

The basic values, principles, and assumptions of western medicine and bioethics are themselves historically situated and culturally determined. '... what has been a professional and expert-driven exercise now needs to incorporate patients' views. The authority over dying must now be invested in patients. Patients' concepts of a good death should guide our efforts to make deaths better' (Clark 2003:174). In view of the emphasis on patient-centred care, it is important to go deeper and find out patients' and relatives' conceptions of a good death so that everyone, regardless of religion or culture, can die a dignified death congruent with his/her world view.

References

Aspinall P (2000) 'Ethnic Groups and Our healthier nation: whither the informa- tion age?' *Journal of Public Health Medicine* 21:2:125–32.

Blakemore K (2000) 'Health and social care needs in minority communities: an over-problemetized issue?' *Health and Social Care in the Community* 8(1):22–30.

Blakemore K and Boneham M (1994) *Age Race and Ethnicity a Comparative Approach.* Open University Press, Buckingham.

Bowes A and Domakos T (1995) 'Key issues in South Asian women's health: a study in Glasgow. *Social Sciences in Health* 1:3:145–57.

Boyle D (1998) 'The cultural context of dying from cancer'. *International Journal of Palliative Nursing* (2): 70–83.

CEEHD (2003) 'Concepts of Diversity', The Centre for Evidence in Ethnicity, Health and Diversity, Website.

Chattoo S, Ahmad W, Haworth M, and Lennard R (2002) *South Asian and White Patients with Advanced Cancer: Patients' and Families' Experiences of the Illness and Perceived Needs for Care* (Final Report to CRC UK and the DoH), Centre for Research in Primary Care, University of Leeds.

Choudhury P (1999) *Comparison of Uptake of Specialist Palliative Care Services by Asian Patients and White Patients in Wolverhampton,* unpublished MMedSci Thesis, Keele University.

Chibnall J, Videen S, Duckro P, and Miller D (2002) 'Psychosocial-spiritual correlates of death distress in patients with life-threatening medical conditions'. *Palliative Medicine* 16:331–8.

Clark J (2003) 'Patient centred death'. *BMJ*, **327**:174–5.

Coup A (1996) 'Cultural safety and culturally congruent care: a comparative analysis of Irhapeti Ramsden's and Madeleine Leininger's educational projects for practice', *Nursing Praxis in New Zealand*, March 11 (1) 4–11.

Erwin J and Peters B (1999) 'Treatment issues for HIV Africans in London'. *Social Science and Medicine* **49**:1519–28.

Firth S (1997) *Dying, Death and Bereavement in a British Hindu Community*. Peeters, Leuven.

Firth S (2001) *Wider Horizons: Care of the Dying in a Multicultural Society*, National Council for Hospice and Specialist Palliative Care Services, London.

Gardner K (2002) *Age, Narrative and Migration: The Life Course and Life Histories of Bangladeshi Elders in London*. Berg, Oxford.

Gatrad A, Brown E, Notta H, and Sheikh A (2003) 'Palliative care needs of minorities'. *BMJ*, **327**:176–7.

Gerrish K (1999) 'Inequalities in service provision: an examination of institutional influences on the provision of district nursing care to minority ethnic communities'. *Journal of Advanced Nursing* **30**:**6**:1263–71, Dec. 30.

Gerrish K, Husband C and Mackenzie J (1996) *Nursing for a Multi-ethnic Society*. Open University Press, Buckingham.

Gilliat-Ray S (2001) 'Sociological Perspectives on the Pastoral Care of Minority Faiths in Hospital'. In Orchard H (ed.) *Spirituality in Health Care Contexts*, pp. 135–46. Jessica Kingsley, London.

Gunaratnam Y (2003) *Researching 'Race' and Ethnicity: Methods, Knowledge and Power*. Sage, London.

Gunaratnam Y, Bremner I, Pollock L, and Weir C (1998) 'Anti-discrimination, emotions and professional practice'. *European Journal of Palliative Care* **5**(4), 122–6.

Harding S and Rosato M (1999) 'Cancer incidence among first generation Scottish, Irish, West Indian and South Asian Migrants living in England and Wales'. *Ethnicity and Health* 1999, 491/2, 83–92.

Johnson M, Bains J, Chaunban J, Saleem B, and Tomlins R (2001) *Palliative Care, Cancer and a Literature Review*, Report to the Birmingham Specialist Community Health NHS Trust and Macmillan Cancer Relief, Ashram Agency and De Montfort University.

Jones K (2003) *Diversities in Approach to End-of-Life: a View from Britain of the Qualitative Literature*. Centre for Evidence in Ethnicity, Health & Diversity, Mary Seacole Research Centre, DeMontfort University.

Kagawa-Singer M and Blackhall L (2001*)* 'Negotiating cross-cultural issues at the end of life: "You got to go where he lives"'. *Journal of the American Medical Association* **286**:2993–3001.

Karim K, Bailey M, and Tunna K (2000) 'Non-white ethnicity and the provision of specialist palliative care services: factors affecting doctors' referral patterns'. *Palliative Medicine* 2000:14:471–8.

Katz J (2000) 'Jewish perspectives on death, dying and bereavement'. In Dickenson D, Johnson M, and Katz J (ed.) *Death, Dying and Bereavement*. Open University and Sage, London.

Koffman J and Higginson I (2001) 'Accounts of carers' satisfaction with health care at the end of life: a comparison of first generation black Caribbeans and white patients with advanced disease'. *Palliative Medicine* 15(4):337–45.

Krakauer E, Crenner C, and Fox K (2002) Barriers to optimum end-of-life care for minority patients'. *Journal of the American Geriatrics Society* 50:182–90.

Lie A (2001) 'No level playing field: the multifaith context and its challenges'. In Orchard H (ed.) *Spirituality in Health Care Contexts*, pp. 183–93. Jessica Kingsley, London.

Lund S (2002) 'An exploration of the palliative care needs of the Asian community in Slough', Health related research fellowship, Final Report, 2000–2002, Reading University.

National Council (2003) *Studies on Chinese community experience of cancer care*. Information Exchange No 37, October, London, National Council for Hospice and Specialist Palliative Care Services, p. 10.

Ng L, Schumacher A, and Goh C (2000) 'Autonomy for whom? A perspective from the Orient'. *Palliative Medicine* 14:163–64.

Orchard H (ed.) (2001) *Spirituality in Health Care Contexts*. Jessica Kingsley, London.

Orchard H (2001) 'Being There? Presence and Absence in Spiritual Care Delivery'. In Orchard (ed.) *Spirituality in Health Care Contexts*, pp. 147–59. Jessica Kingsley, London.

Papadopoulos I, Tilki M, and Taylor G (1998) *Transcultural Care: A Guide for Health Care Professionals*. Quay Books, Salisbury.

Pfeffer N and Moynihan K (1996) 'Ethnicity and health beliefs with respect to cancer: a critical review of methodology'. *British Journal of Cancer* 74 Suppl. XXIX:S66–S72.

Randhawa G, Owens A, Fitches R, and Khan Z (2003) 'Communication in the development of culturally competent palliative care services in the UK: a case study'. *International Journal of Palliative Nursing* 9:41:24–31.

Shaw A(2000) *'Kinship and Continuity: Pakistani Families in Britain'*. Harwood Academic Press, Amsterdam.

Silvera M and Kapasi K (2000) *'Health Advocacy for Minority Ethnic Londoners: Putting Services on the map?'* King's Fund/NHS Executive, London.

Simmonds R, Sque M, Goddard G, Tullett R, and Mount J (2001) *Improving Access to Palliative Care Services of Ethnic Minority Groups:* a Report of a study funded by the Community Fund. St. Catherine's Hospice, Crawley.

Somerville J (2001) 'The experience of informal carers within the bangladeshi Community'. *International Journal of Palliative Nursing* 7(5):240–7.

Spruyt O (1999) 'Community-based palliative care for Bangladeshi patients in East London: accounts of bereaved carers'. *Palliative Medicine* 13:119–29.

Tse C, Chhong A, and Fok S (2003) 'Breaking bad news'. *Palliative Medicine* 17:339–43.

Tilki M (1998) 'The health of the Irish in Britain'. In Papadopoulos *et al.* (ed.) *Transcultural Care : A Guide for Health Care Professionals*, pp.136–62. Quay Books, Salisbury.

Webb L, Erica Y, Finnegan T, and Siddat M (2000) *No Exclusion Clause: Opening Doors to Better Palliative Care Services for People from a Culturally Diverse Community*, Warwickshire Health Authority.

Werth J, Blevins D, Toussaint K, and Durham M (2002) 'The influence of cultural diversity on end-of-life care and decisions'. *American Behavioural Scientist* 46:2:204–19.

Wright M (2001) 'Chaplaincy in hospice and hospital: findings from a survey in England and Wales'. *Palliative Medicine* 15:229–42.

4

Sexual identity—gender and sexual orientation

Katherine Cox

In this chapter I explore sexual identity as an issue of social difference in relation to death, dying, and bereavement. Gender is a very visible 'difference'; a core aspect of our identity and relationships. Our sexuality is key to our self-understanding and social role but is a private, hidden aspect of ourselves that we may choose, or not, to share with others. Our gendered and sexual roles carry particular social meanings, and social expectations and norms may or may not validate our experiences.

I explore the concept of masculinity and grief to suggest that dying and bereaved men as instrumental grievers (Martin and Doka 2000) are a disenfranchised group both in terms of social expectations and within palliative care provision. I then explore the experience of gay men and lesbians within palliative care to argue that these groups are also disenfranchised within particular socio-cultural norms of what it means to experience loss. In both sections I argue that a more open and flexible response is required from practitioners to allow people their unique experience given their social context.

Gender and palliative care—are men a disenfranchised group in palliative care and bereavement services?

The rise of feminism has brought about a destabilizing of patriarchal values as an unquestioned norm and has given the experience of women an unprecedented voice and status. Gender, as the social elaboration of biological sex differences (Field *et al.* 1997), has become a key factor in our construction of knowledge itself. Unusually, the reverse has been the case in the literature on palliative care. Early bereavement research used interviews with women only (Parkes 1972; Bowlby 1981) yet the results were generalized as universally applicable, and bereavement care has set a feminized reaction to grief as a 'gold standard' against which men's grief is judged (Williams 1998). Recently there has been renewed interest in the experience of men facing bereavement in an attempt to redress this imbalance. This has not been matched however by a corresponding body of literature on the masculine experience of dying.

Men facing life-threatening conditions

Just as bereavement can be understood as a crisis which needs to be faced with all the arsenal of coping strategies at one's disposal, so dying can be understood as perhaps the greatest challenge and crisis any of us has to face. When the 'fight it, beat it, lick it' language of curative medicine is no longer applicable, a man facing a terminal prognosis must adapt to face this qualitatively different challenge. He may not experience an affective response of despair and loss but he may need assistance and encouragement actively to engage in the process, to make concrete choices about how he wishes to live his life, where he wishes to die, what treatments he will accept, and with whom he wishes to spend time. The use of denial and the role of hope may be important. We must ensure that we do not emasculate a man facing terminal illness—he should be given choices and control and remain at the centre of any decision-making.

The double bind of contemporary masculinity

Traditionally, men are expected to be in control, rational, analytical, assertive, courageous, and fulfilling a protector and provider role (Lund 2001). At the same time, the rise of feminism and 'New Man' culture gives rise to an expectation that men should be emotionally expressive, sensitive and gentle. Men facing death or bereavement will be doing so within this very particular socio-cultural double bind.

It is important to bear in mind two caveats. We must acknowledge the vast variety of response within gender groups; the arguments presented here can only be very broad generalizations. Different ways of grieving are related to but not tied to gender (Martin and Doka 2000). It is also important to remember the presence of other differentials such as age, point in the lifespan, sexuality, type of loss, ethnicity, and social class. Gender is only one of an array of social and psychological factors that will influence our attitudes to death, dying, and bereavement.

Do men and women deal differently with death and bereavement?

It is now generally understood that men and women grieve differently (Stroebe *et al.* 1993; Lund 2001). Men show less acceptance of the death, become involved sooner in romantic relationships, express themselves less, and consume more alcohol. Other studies demonstrate increase in health problems for widowers and increased mortality rates, particularly through suicide, compared with widows (ibid). The loss of a partner results in a more significant decrease in social support for widowers than for widows; men are more likely to be socially isolated and less likely to express their feelings; widowers may feel a greater need than widows to return to work; men use self-help groups less, and are more private, intellectual and introspective in their grief. Gender differences in conjugal bereavement in part arise from differences in the roles that had been filled by the surviving partners' spouse, for example cleaning, shopping, and cooking, although generational factors also affect these results. Men's greater vulnerability may stem in part from the fact that they may have depended on their wives to maintain relationships outside the family, both with friends and with adult children.

These differences, arising from the different ways in which men and women function in terms of their social relationships and social roles, have given rise to a controversial debate about the efficacy of men's grieving patterns and the pattern of responses from bereavement care services. Other studies, however, note a *lack* of gender differences in long-term bereavement outcome (Lund 2001). What this points to is that, although the style of grief may be different for men and for women, the end result in terms of health and functioning will be the same, which suggests that there is no qualitatively 'better' way to grieve.

Other writers (Williams 1998) have questioned the use of gender comparison given that many women will grieve in a traditionally 'male' way and vice versa and call instead for the development of 'models of diversity'. Comparison risks perpetuating hierarchized positions and gender polarization, whereas an openness to diversity creates a richer potential for both men and women. There are, however, very real differences in the social construction of gender roles, as the following case studies illustrate. In order to create a more open response to difference, we must first increase our awareness of those differences by exploring them in a spirit of openness.

Case Study A

Peter is a thirty-five year old man whose wife, Ellen, is dying from bowel cancer. They have three young children. Whilst Ellen has benefited from counselling and the local cancer support group, Peter has politely evaded any offer of emotional support. He works hard at his job as a retail manager and at caring for the children and is clearly devoted to his wife. He plays football regularly.

Case Study B

Henry is a thirty-eight year old man with pancreatic cancer. He is an accountant, a keen cricketer, married with a seven year old son, Hugo. He was admitted to the hospice because his wife, Mary, said she could no longer cope with his angry and aggressive outbursts. After discussion with the doctor about his prognosis, Henry decided to make a will, plan his funeral, and give Hugo his cricket bat signed by the England team. He and Hugo do not speak much but they read stories together and play cricket out on the grass, Henry teaching Hugo to bowl.

Masculinity and ontological security

The emotions commonly associated with loss and grief do not sit comfortably with a traditional masculine role and can present men with a destabilizing experience, undermining their sense of who they are and how they function in their social relationships. Sickness or bereavement may threaten a masculine sense of ontological security, breaking down the individual's taken-for-granted relationship with the social world (Thompson in Lund 2001), precipitating a profound state of crisis.

Dual-process model

Stroebe and Schut (1995) argue that grief can be understood according to a dual-process model—a dialectic of 'blended grief' which is held in a different balance for different people at different times. On the one hand there is an orientation to loss; a need to express emotion, to feel the extent of the grief and actively mourn—intuitive grief. On the other there is an orientation towards restoration; an instrumental aspect to grief which is concerned with practical coping tasks, concrete concerns, and looking to the future. This has given rise to a consideration of gender differences in the light of this model (Martin and Doka 2000); are men instrumental grievers and, if so, is this as effective a grief response as intuitive grieving? Is it simply that men may experience this dynamic in a different balance from women? This model can also be applied to men facing life-threatening conditions. Men who are dying will experience the relationship between an affective response to the illness and a need to cope in a concrete way with the situation, and will experience this perhaps with a particular emphasis on the need to cope.

In supporting someone in crisis, it is more effective to use an approach which supports their existing coping style rather than impose a set of coping strategies which feel jarring and unfamiliar. If an intuitive style of grieving is a more typically female response to bereavement and an instrumental style a more typical male response, palliative care services need to support and sustain both. On the other hand, 'blended grievers' (Martin and Doka 2000) may hold both styles in a particular relationship. These models of grief are equally applicable for people facing the crisis of terminal illness.

A critique of palliative care and bereavement services

Case Study A

In the hospice ward round, concern is expressed about Peter who is felt to be 'in denial' and obstructing the offers of counselling. Staff report that they have repeatedly offered Peter the opportunity to talk about his feelings but he evades the issue. He is felt to be 'at risk' in terms of his long-term coping.

Case Study B

Ward staff are also concerned about Henry who is planning a holiday with his wife, even though his prognosis is short. He also is regarded as being 'in denial'.

Psycho-social palliative care and bereavement services traditionally emphasize the expression of emotion, a requirement both to feel and express loss and grief. This approach may simply not be appropriate for some men (nor for some women). In the face of pressure to feel and express emotion in a particular way, grieving men are disenfranchised by services and by a wider cultural imperative towards affective expression. Men may be dissonant grievers (Martin and Doka 2000) in that the way they experience grief may clash with a social imperative towards emotional expression. We need to be aware of diversity in gendered response; the potential exclusion of men from intuitively biased bereavement services and the need for gender appropriate services for ill and bereaved men.

'Big boys don't cry'

Case Study A

Peter is in the family room doing a jigsaw puzzle. The social worker sits with Peter and they do the puzzle together. Peter, concentrating on the puzzle, says 'Ellen is the centre of my life. Help me to hold onto the pieces when she dies' The social worker agrees that she will help him to hold onto the pieces. Together they finish the puzzle.

Case Study B

One of the nurses joins Henry and Hugo who are playing cricket out on the grass. She fields whilst Hugo bowls to Henry who is batting from his wheelchair.

Social norms and gender expectations not only influence how emotions are expressed but also how they are understood and felt (Field *et al.* 1997). Many men express their loss *through* an instrumental focus; they may not cry and express grief affectively, not because they are repressing those feelings but because they construct their grief response in terms of active coping and practical tasks. If so, it is at this level that they can best be supported. A grieving man is better served if he is given the space, permission, and resources to express his grief consistent with his understanding of himself and his social role.

What can help terminally ill and bereaved men?

Palliative care services need to focus on strategies and networks, formal and informal, which will enable men to cope with the crisis of illness and bereavement. This will involve assisting the man to develop an internal locus of control, a sense of self-efficacy, building on his prior history of coping and his self-esteem (Lund 2001):

Practical coping

Case Study A

After Ellen's death, Peter worked out how he could return to work by asking his parents-in-law to take the children after school. On the advice of another single parent at work, he talked to his employer about working more flexible hours to incorporate child care.

Case Study B

Mary decides that she will leave Hugo and Henry alone together for a portion of each day. They play outside or with lego in the children's room. Henry teaches Hugo how to pump up the tyres in his wheelchair and Hugo pushes his dad around the unit with great pride.

Older men facing the loss of a wife may have to cope with secondary losses such as the loss of housekeeper, cook etc. which may undermine their ability to cope with the practical tasks of daily living. Younger men experiencing bereavement may have to cope with single parenthood. Men facing terminal illness will have to cope with loss of physical effectiveness, loss of role in employment and in the family, loss of future.

Grief may be both expressed *and felt* through these very practical challenges and the path through grief is in rising to those challenges. Practically based support groups may assist with information sharing and assistance with coping styles as well as create a community of support.

Sex and remarriage

For some men, sex and sexual activity is an important, life-affirming aspect of their lives and will therefore be crucial in coping after a bereavement. For some, remarriage is an important aspect of coping after the loss of a wife, in order to have a sexual relationship and/or for companionship, support and practical assistance with daily living. For men facing terminal illness, private time with their partner and the opportunity for physical closeness may be very valuable.

Case Study B

Once Henry is in the hospice, Mary feels more free to relax with her husband. Some nights she arranges for Hugo to stay with her parents and she sleeps on the unit with Henry.

Social contact

One of the most significant factors in bereavement outcome for men lies in the depth and range of attachments. For widowers these are often largely sustained by the wife and, after her death, her spouse may be left isolated and lacking the experience and skills to form and maintain relationships

(Walter 1999). Bereaved men may require specific information, support and encouragement to make and maintain social contacts with other bereaved people, friends, colleagues, and family members. Men facing terminal illness may also need to be encouraged to maintain social contact.

Case Study B

Henry had refused to see his friends on the cricket team, he said it would be too depressing. Finally, on his birthday, he agreed that they could visit. The hospice staff made a cake and gave everyone a beer and the atmosphere was relaxed and easy.

Generative activity

Many men consider it important to maintain a role in the world with an attendant sense of purpose and efficacy. This may be provided through employment, voluntary work, helping with grandchildren, participating in community work or further education.

Case Study A

Frank, Ellen's father, looks after his three young grandchildren twice a week. He cooks their meal, plays with them, helps with their homework. On fishing trips with his youngest grandson he tells stories about Ellen when she was a girl.

Books and online resources

Written information can be very helpful as a solitary activity in which the person remains in control of the amount of information they access at any one time. Palliative care services should have a library of resources that they can make available to their clients (e.g. Bly 1990; Keen 1991; Golden and Miller 1998).

Counselling

Case Study A

Peter did not want counselling. The conversations he had with the social worker focused on what he was thinking rather than how he was feeling and what he could practically do to cope with the situation.

Men need to have their pattern of grieving validated and respected. Counsellors need to be able to assess the person's coping style, identify boundaries to the person's method of coping response and enable the person to live through their experience in the way most appropriate for them.

One-to-one support can be usefully framed in terms of problem solving and action with the emphasis on cognitive processing and concrete behaviour. Logical analysis, cognitive restructuring, cognitive avoidance or denial, information seeking, and behavioural monitoring provide an appropriate rationale for this type of approach (Williams 1998; Martin and Doka 2000; Lund 2001).

Enabling men to explore safe ways of expressing emotion can be a valuable tool. Channelling anger into concrete and affirmative action in a rational and thought-focused way might be methods by which a man can express destabilizing and intense affect in ways which give him back some measure of control and efficacy. Channels for expression that feel acceptable: going to a football match, political action, playing music, telling stories, writing etc. may enable him to express difficult feelings in ways which do not threaten his identity. Practical tasks such as writing a will, planning for the family's future or, for a bereaved man, making a memorial stone, visiting the cemetery etc. may in themselves be healing (Lund 2001).

Groups

Case Study B

Henry spends time in the smoking area with Spencer, a 60-year-old man with a brain tumour. Whilst they talk little about their illness, they swap stories about sport and watch the football together. On the night that Spencer dies, Henry sat with him, holding his hand.

Men have traditionally distanced themselves from support group services and any group support may need to take men's specific needs into account (Williams 1996). Men can help one another simply by being together (Lund 2001) without necessarily talking in depth about their experiences. A less formally structured group allowing for social activities, practical problem-solving and plenty of opportunity for humour may fit the requirements of bereaved men better than a formal support group. Encouraging men to participate in leisure and community-based activities may provide a supportive forum outside formal bereavement services.

Family and couple support

Different styles of grieving may generate stress and tension within a family. Bereavement services should aim to enable different family members to recognize the strengths in each other's grieving styles and to validate each other's response.

How strict is the gender divide in grieving styles?

Although grieving styles are related to gender there are many exceptions to general patterns. A different challenge is presented to the man whose grief is experienced as intense emotional affect, who is overwhelmed by the loss and who requires a space and the means to express the intensity of his feeling. He may benefit from the 'talking therapy' of traditional bereavement counselling as well as reassurance about his ability to cope and to function in the long term. Conversely, a woman whose grief pattern is instrumental will require validation and recognition of the legitimacy of her response.

Case Study A

Teachers are concerned that Ellen's seven year old daughter Holly is 'in denial' as her behaviour seems unaffected by events at home. Holly does not cry over her mother's death and she resists attempts made by the school welfare officer to talk about her feelings. Every evening she writes a letter to her mother in her journal and every weekend she takes flowers to her mother's grave.

Palliative care and bereavement services need to be open to and respectful of different ways of coping with illness and bereavement and the ways in which gender as a social construction will affect grief response. Men have traditionally been excluded from bereavement care services (Williams 1997) and are still excluded from the literature on palliative care. We must acknowledge the diverse ways in which men meet the challenge of terminal illness and loss. We need to listen with respect and humility to the experience of the individual whilst holding an understanding of the social construction of gender roles. In opening up our perspective, we free up the possibilities for women as much as for men (Williams 1998).

Sexual orientation and palliative care—gay men and lesbians and their partners facing life-threatening conditions

In this section I explore the impact of sexual orientation for gay men and lesbians in palliative care and bereavement services. Whilst the emotional impact of living with a life-threatening condition may be similar across different communities, the social context in which those feelings are experienced will markedly affect their psychological impact. I look at the research context; the need to consider sexuality in the provision of holistic care; the impact of homophobia; the implications for practice in terms of the practical and social issues faced by lesbian and gay patients and their partners and the potential emotional impact of social exclusion as a result of sexual orientation.

The research context

There is a significant lack of research concerning the specific experiences of lesbians and gay men in palliative care services. The literature on sexuality and health care from a heterosexual perspective (e.g. Field *et al.* 1997; Oliviere *et al.* 1998) is a welcome contribution to the field in that it acknowledges the importance of considering sex and sexuality in the provision of holistic care but does not consider the particular experience of lesbians and gay men.

The literature on palliative care for gay men with HIV (e.g. Sherr 1995; Fisher *et al.* 1996; Kellerhouse 1996) can in many ways translate to the experience of lesbians and gay men facing or affected by other life-threatening conditions but there is no literature which takes account of the differences. HIV is a specific social experience carrying a specific social weight. Lesbians and gay men with other life-threatening conditions will have a qualitatively different experience. This literature dates from a period when most gay men with AIDS had a very short prognosis. The fact that the context is now one of prolonged prognosis and better health will potentially exclude gay men dying as a result of HIV, not only from society in general but from the gay and the HIV positive communities where HIV is no longer regarded by many as a terminal condition.

Lesbians and gay men using bereavement care services will experience *disenfranchised loss*. Doka (1989) suggests that disenfranchised loss has a paradox at its heart: the very nature of this type of grief exacerbates the problems of grief, but the usual sources of support may not be available or helpful. Grief may be disenfranchised because the relationship is not recognized and therefore the loss is not recognized. Lesbians and gay men using palliative care services do so within a general social context of exclusion.

The role of sexuality in holistic care

All of us are sexual beings and our sexuality is an integral part of us, whether we are or are not sexually active (Oliviere *et al.* 1998). Sexuality is much more than the biological aspect of sex and is also more all-encompassing than the emotional aspect of sexual relationships, it is a core aspect of our social identity and our relationships. So if sexuality is integral to palliative care, are we meeting the needs of lesbians and gay men?

Whilst lesbians and gay men are as heterogeneous a group as any other, they are connected by a history of social difficulties. This history and the context in which many gay men and lesbians currently live their lives is one of homophobia and social exclusion.

The impact of homophobia in palliative care services

Homophobic prejudice potentially affects both staff and patients in palliative care through heterosexism—covert discrimination through an assumption of heterosexuality, and homophobia—overt prejudice against gay men, lesbians, and bisexuals. So far no legal protection exists against homophobia in the workplace which makes it even more important that it is addressed as a specific issue within the policies and culture of the organization.

Staff issues—sexual orientation in the hospice

How we feel about ourselves as sexual beings and how we function as a team in this area has a direct impact on the care we give patients and those close to them. Issues for hospice staff working with lesbians and gay men may include unresolved feelings in ourselves about sex and sexual preference or embarrassment over irrational responses. No-one approaches this issue neutrally, everyone will bring their own experiences, feelings, views, and biases; when we are aware of our own feelings we are better able to attune to our patients' feelings.

Case Study

Fiona is admitted to the hospice with advanced metastatic breast cancer. She is accompanied by her partner Sarah. The doctor clerking her in asks about next of kin and, turning to Fiona says, 'You're her daughter I presume?' A lesbian nurse, who is not open about her sexuality at work, overhears the remark and considers the implications for herself in challenging the doctor about his assumption.

Implications for practice

1. Practical issues

There are concrete ways in which we can assist gay men and lesbians facing life-threatening conditions in promoting and securing their rights and wishes within a social context of exclusion.

(a) Wills

Case Study

Gordon and John had been together for 10 years when John died suddenly. His parents as the legal next of kin made all the funeral arrangements without including Gordon. They inherited half of the house and so Gordon lost his home as well as half of all his jointly owned possessions.

If a person dies intestate, their estate is divided up under the rules of intestacy and a same sex partner has no legal claim. A lesbian or gay man wishing to leave their possessions to their partner must make their wishes clear in a will.

(b) Living wills

Case Study

Steve was suffering from HIV related dementia and was unable to make treatment decisions for himself. Jake and Steve had been together for many years but in the absence of blood family the HIV consultant insisted that she made the decisions on Steve's behalf.

A Living Will, or Advance Directive is a set of advance instructions from a person of sound mind about their future medical care e.g. refusal or acceptance of treatments. This is not legally binding in the UK but most doctors will respect the wishes written in a living will. Unless a living will has been made, the family of origin can make decisions about medical intervention regardless of how long a gay or lesbian couple have been together. In a Living Will the patient can specify a named person who they want to make decisions on their behalf should the need arise. This is another important means by which the role of the patient's partner can be validated.

(c) Power of attorney

A lesbian or gay man can designate a partner or friend to act on their behalf if they become mentally incapable. Otherwise, this right passes directly to the legal next of kin.

2. Social issues

Lesbians and gay men facing life-threatening conditions or who have been bereaved live through these experiences within a particular social context.

(a) Lack of recognition and exclusion

Social norms specify who can grieve, how much, for how long, and in what way. Those who have lost a same sex partner are not accorded the same rights and privileges in the expression of grief as heterosexual partners. There is a connection between being given permission and giving oneself permission to grieve. Bereaved lesbians and gay men may themselves struggle to recognize the full extent of their loss when they receive no validation from others. Health care practitioners are in a unique position to validate and respect 'disenfranchised' loss and to provide bereaved same sex partners with a safe space to have their grief heard and acknowledged.

(b) Secrecy

People may be unable to say at work or to friends/family that their same sex partner has died. When a heterosexual spouse dies, the surviving partner has a recognized social role of widow/er which carries social status and legal and social rights; bereaved spouses may have time off work, apply for benefit, they are excused certain social responsibilities and permitted a wider range of emotional expression. All of these may be denied a same sex partner.

(c) Partner/family

Whilst lesbian and gay communities are in no way monolithic, for many the gay and lesbian community is their 'family' of choice. We need to question, broaden and revise our idea of family in the provision of bereavement care.

In many cases there is a good relationship between a lesbian or gay partner and family and they can provide an important support for each other. In other cases the relationship is a source of stress and conflict. People may be forced at the point of illness to tell their families they are lesbian or gay, or may choose never to disclose their sexual orientation which can cause stress and confusion after death.

Many gay men distance themselves both geographically and emotionally from their parents and bridging the gap can be challenging for all parties. Sometimes only certain family members know and family secrets can cause even more distress. Parents may feel anger at their child's sexuality especially if they feel it has contributed to their child's death, and if they learn about both at the same time, the two are more likely to be conflated. As mourners they also will be stigmatized; parents who may be homophobic will themselves become the target of homophobic prejudice. Their anger can then easily be projected on the surviving partner.

(d) Funerals

Funerals are significant spaces within which the deceased person's sexuality and bereaved partner/friends can be publicly validated. Acknowledging all aspects of the person's life and all their relationships can, however, present a significant challenge. Families may forbid the partner from attending the service, and refuse to disclose the nature of the death to relatives if it was the result of AIDS. Palliative care workers may be able to play an important part in assisting family and partner to reach a consensus in making funeral plans. Alternatively, they may assist same sex partners in developing other rituals which might give a sense of validation and closure.

(e) Multiple loss

The concept of bereavement overload (Kastenbaum in Fiegal 1977) is applicable to many gay men in relation to losses associated with HIV. Research has found a direct relationship between the number of bereavements and symptoms of post-traumatic stress response, demoralization, sleep problems, sedative use, recreational drug use, use of psychology services, and suicide (O'Brien 1992; Sherr 1995; Sherr et al. 1996). When providing bereavement support, we must be aware that the social and historical context of the loss may have a significant effect on the bereaved person.

3. The emotional impact of social exclusion

(a) Lesbian experience

Case Study

Mary is a forty year old woman who has been caring for her ex-husband at home prior to his admission. Whilst he is in the hospice she visits him with their ten year old son and they are clearly still very close. She talks evasively to the social worker about problems at home with her new partner. It is only when the worker specifically allows the possibility that her partner is a woman that she is able to talk about the pressures on this new relationship given the fact that she has returned to care for her husband. She had been afraid to disclose because of her son and because she was afraid for her career as a nursery nurse. After having both her ongoing bond with her ex-husband and her lesbian relationship validated, she was able to visit with her partner and they both felt less excluded and marginalized.

Lesbian women will have to cope with the fear of social, institutional and medical prejudice when accessing health care. This may mean that a lesbian may present far later and perhaps be more anxious about the quality of the treatment she will receive; whether her definition of her family will be respected and whether appropriate social and psychological support will be available for her and significant others.

As is so often the case when issues of sexual orientation are considered, the voice of lesbians is silenced or simply 'tagged on' to gay men's issues when in fact lesbian experience will be qualitatively different both from heterosexual women and gay men. Lesbian women may well have children to consider and may be afraid that disclosure will jeopardise wishes for future child care arrangements. Health care professionals may be more aware of the needs of gay men as a result of HIV but may demonstrate a marked lack of awareness of the needs of lesbian patients and partners. The almost complete lack of literature on this subject and of services specifically for lesbian women indicate their continued oppression through silence.

(b) Loss of looks and loss of sexual activity/function

The changes associated with illness and bereavement can have a significant impact on a person's social, political, and sexual identity. Changes in the physical self can threaten a person's sense of belonging in the gay community with its emphasis on youth, beauty, and health. Loss of sexual activity/function through illness or bereavement can undermine the individual's identity as a gay man or lesbian.

(c) Relationships

For an HIV positive man, watching someone die as a result of HIV may evoke powerful identification with the dying person and grief itself can suppress immune function (Colburn and Malena 1988; O'Brien 1992). HIV positive men may experience survival guilt and adjusting to an identity as a gay man living with HIV or as a single gay bereaved man after the loss of a partner involves significant change in identity and role. HIV positive men must face the additional impact of the virus on forming and maintaining relationships, or cope with the lack of relationship. Living out these complexities can be even harder within the social context of a sexualized urban gay culture.

(d) Mental health issues

Young gay men are at a far higher risk of suicide than other members of the population and statistically show a far higher use of mental health services (Sherr *et al.* 1998). We must be aware of the particular emotional and psychological impact for gay men and lesbians of facing a life-threatening condition or of losing their partner, given the other social stresses which will be impacting on them.

(e) Religious and spiritual issues

Many gay men and lesbians will find themselves on the fringe or outside their particular religious communities and are not able to draw on the very source of support they need in their grief. Religious leaders have an important role in countering the religious guilt people often feel in relation to their sexuality.

(f) Bereavement care

Bereavement counsellors working with lesbians and gay men should use theories of grief which avoid generalized applications and allow greater scope for individual experience. We must be aware of the specific impact of the loss of a same sex partner, a gay or lesbian friend, or a gay or lesbian family member may have on the person grieving. People need to have the opportunity to talk through their pain in a sensitive, compassionate, understanding, and respectful environment which validates the relationship. People need to be seen and to see themselves as worthy of support. Particularly if people are not able to speak of their bereavement publicly, at work, or if their loss is not acknowledged by their own family or the deceased's family, it is important that they have somewhere that their pain is acknowledged and heard.

Meeting needs of lesbians and gay men

♦ Palliative care services need to address issues of homophobia at policy level, in the team's functioning and in the context of staff training and education. Concrete measures must be taken to ensure that these issues are addressed in an ongoing and constructive way through monitoring and assessment.

♦ Palliative care services must be aware of the social, historical, and sexual context within which a patient accesses the service.

♦ Palliative care services must ensure that specific information is given to lesbian and gay patients about the implications of Wills, Advance Directives, and appointing a Power of Attorney.

♦ Bereavement services must consider the social context of lesbians and gay men and offer particular support for those whose loss is disenfranchised because of sexual orientation.

Conclusion—Death and dying in a postmodern world

There is a loss of gendered and sexual certainties over how to die and how to mourn. Our particular project in a post-modern world is to construct a path for ourselves out of a range of possibilities. We have lost the grand narrative and have now to position ourselves in relation to an overwhelming choice of ways to be (Field *et al.* 1997). Those of us working within the field of palliative care and bereavement services need to understand the social context within which our clients live their individual gendered and sexual lives. Men and women, gay, lesbian, bisexual, and heterosexual, we need to rise to this unique challenge of our time and write our own stories.

References

Bly R (1990) *Iron John: A Book About Men.* Vintage, New York.

Bowlby J (1981) *Loss, Sadness and Depression.* Penguin, Harmondsworth.

Colburn K and Malena D(1988) 'Bereavement issues for survivors of persons with AIDS: coping with society's pressures' *Hospice Care* 9/10.

Doka K (ed.) (1989) *Disenfranchised Grief: Recognising Hidden Sorrow.* Lexington Books, Massachusetts.

Fiegal H (ed.) (1977) *New Meanings of Life.* McGraw-Hill, New York.

Field D, Hockey J, and Small N (ed.)(1997) *Death, Gender and Ethnicity.* Routledge, London.

Fisher A, Vohr F, and Wacker M (1996) 'Role of in-hospital palliative care service'. *XI International Conference on AIDS, Geneva,* May.

Golden T and Miller J (1998) *When a Man Faces Grief.* Willowgreen, Indiana.

Keen S (1991) *Fire in the Belly: on Being a Man.* Bantam, New York.

Kellerhouse B (1996) 'Voices from the front: the consequences of AIDS-related loss on six HIV negative gay men living in New York city'. *XI International Conference on AIDS, Geneva,* May.

Lund D (ed.)(2001) *Men Coping with Grief.* Baywood, New York.

Martin T and Doka K (2000) *Men Don't Cry...Women Do: Transcending Gender Stereotypes of Grief.* Taylor and Francis, Philadelphia.

O'Brien M (1992) *Living with AIDS: An Experiment in Courage.* Aubern House, London.

Oliviere D, Hargreaves R, and Monroe B (1998) *Good Practices in Palliative Care: A Psychosocial Perspective.* Ashgate, Aldershot.

Parkes CM (1972) *Bereavement: Studies of Grief in Adult Life.* Penguin, Harmondsworth.

Sherr L (ed.) (1995) *Grief and AIDS.* John Wiley & Sons, Chichester.

Sherr L, Campbell N, Crosier A, and Meldrum J (1996) 'Suicide and AIDS: A Report of the European Initiative'. *XI International Conference on AIDS, Geneva,* May.

Stroebe M and Schut H (1995) 'Sex differences in bereavement'. *Progress in Palliative Care* 4:85–7.

Stroebe M, Stroebe W, and Hansson R (1993, 1994) *Handbook of Bereavement: Theory, Research and Intervention.* Cambridge University Press, Cambridge.

Walter T (1999, 2001) *On Bereavement, The Culture of Grief.* Open University Press, Buckingham.

Williams M (1996) 'Men and bereavement: a general hospice survey'. *Newsletter of the National Association of Bereavement Services,* issue 21.

Williams M (1997) 'Making time for the 'hidden' visitors: a study of nurse perceptions of male visitors to a hospice ward'. *Fifth International Congress of Specialist Palliative Care Services,* London, Sept.

Williams M (1998) *Listening to Men's Voices: A Male Perspective on Bereavement.* MSc dissertation, London, St Christopher's Hospice.

5

Older people

Ann McMurray

The aim of this chapter is to examine the concept of ageism in relation to death, dying palliative care services, and older people. Ageism can be described as any attitude, action, or institutional structure that subordinates a person or group because of age or any assignment of roles in society purely on the basis of age. Butler (1969) used the term 'ageism' to describe a stereotypic and negative bias against older people in society. A reflection on the popular culture that exists in health and social care organizations exposes the fact that it perpetuates many negative aspects of ageism. Institutionalized ageism develops either directly, where individuals are treated differently because they are above a certain age or indirectly, where a practice or service has no explicit age bias but still has a disproportionate impact on a particular age group. In the United Kingdom, government legislation has attempted to address ageism in relation to older people. However, organizations continue to demonstrate practices that reinforce ageism and this has an impact on the design and delivery of services.

There is evidence to suggest that older people experience a form of oppression generated by ageism. Research fails to challenge the myths and ideologies that promote ageism in society and older adults are often excluded from the research process. Many organizations positively discriminate in favour of the economically productive. In health and social care, decisions are made about the allocation of resources that covertly deny older people access to services. Institutions such as hospitals reinforce negative stereotyping by focusing on acute services rather than chronic illness and palliative care that is often what older adults need. Age issues are often excluded from the core training of health and social care professionals.

Ageism has consequences. Society has certain expectations about how older people should behave. Older people with palliative care needs may conform to the promoted stereotypes by reducing activity and not seeking appropriate services. The consequences of prejudice can be internalized and as a result generate low self-esteem that can ultimately lead to depression. Older people may present as a socially excluded group, without a voice who are denied services, opportunities, and rights. Old age is viewed by many as the anti-climax of life, associated with non-achievement, loss, and deprivation.

Demography

From the early 1900s life expectancy has increased, influenced by factors such as improved health care. In the year 2000, there were over 10.7 million people of pensionable age in the United Kingdom and this statistic is expected to rise to 12.2 million by 2021. In 1999, figures for England and Wales indicated that 5523 people were aged 100 or more (Age Concern web site 2000). By 2066, it is expected that there will be 95 000 people in this group (ONS 1996).

These statistics have implications for future planning of health and social care services specifically targeted at older people. In the United Kingdom in 2000, 57 per cent of people aged 65–74 and 64 per cent of people over the age of 75 in the General Household Survey reported living with a chronic illness of several years duration. Forty seven per cent said that the illness limited their life style and had implications for their ability to access services. The Alzheimer's Society estimated that 700 000 people in the United Kingdom were living with dementia (Alzheimer's Society website 1997). The chances of having this condition rise sharply with age: 1 in 20 people aged over 65 and 1 in 5 people aged over 80, will develop dementia. These trends need to be incorporated into the planning and provision of palliative care services. Older person households have lower incomes and as such are less able to purchase services. The Department for Works and Pensions estimates that in 1999/2000 between 22 per cent and 36 per cent of older people who were entitled to Income Support did not make a claim (Department for Works and Pensions 1999/2000). The most acute deprivation is experienced by older people living alone who are mainly dependent on State pensions.

Health and social policy

In post-war Britain, a culture developed where the concepts of death and dying were not openly acknowledged. Townsend (1962) provided a graphic insight into the quality of the dying process for older people using experience of nursing home care. During the 1970s the focus seemed to shift to institutional care, marked by a rapid expansion of care home places, to accommodate chronically sick and dying people. Older people entered the care system without a systematic assessment of their needs. In response, government legislation began to focus on improving end of life care. Since 1987, Health Authorities were required to make plans for the provision of palliative care services. However, the reality was that palliative care was regarded as an optional rather than an integral part of the planning process and as such, was given low priority. The NHS and Community Care Act (1990) introduced a code of practice that focused on the specific needs of older people in a variety of care settings including palliative care. The emphasis appeared to shift to the provision of services based on an assessment of need. In reality, service provision was often limited by financial constraints.

Death and dying continued to be absent from the culture of care. The publication of 'A Better Home Life' (Centre for Policy on Ageing 1996), attempted to redress the balance. New policies and procedures were introduced to improve end of life care. The development and expansion of services was further supported by the Care Standards Act (2000), which prepared the way for regulation contained within The Care Homes for Older People: National Minimum Standards (Department of Health 2001a). Furthermore, palliative care was brought onto the national agenda by The NHS Cancer Plan (Department of Health 2000). Specific reference is made to the improving health and social care for older people, eliminating age discrimination, promoting independence in old age, and addressing the palliative care agenda through a government commitment to ensure fairness in funding. The plan set out how improvements in cancer care would be achieved and included the concept of supportive care that would broaden the spectrum of palliative care provision.

The National Service Framework for Older People (Department of Health 2001b), was introduced to address the needs of older people by setting standards across health and social services. The intention was to root out age discrimination and through a single assessment process to match services to the needs of older people. It advocated a palliative care response, which included access to multi-professional teams, and provision of a range of services that addressed the physical, psychological, social, emotional, and spiritual needs of the dying person and their carers. Agencies would be forced to demonstrate that older people were not disadvantaged. In reality, managers found it difficult to implement change. The King's Fund Report issued in response to the National Service Framework recommended a critical assessment of specific services to eliminate policies that disadvantage older people and advocated the implementation of age equality legislation

(Robinson 2002). It recognized that the codes of conduct issued by The General Social Care Council (2003) would ensure that the concept of age discrimination was eliminated from the practice of those employed in social care. Furthermore, the Guidelines on Supportive and Palliative Care issued by the National Institute for Clinical Excellence (2003, Draft) would inform the development of service models for other groups with similar palliative care needs. The Cancer Networks who have a strategic view should build on this work and minimize inequality of access.

Access to palliative care services

Inequalities exist regarding access to palliative care services. The language of palliative care seems to be focused on access to services based on diagnoses rather than need. Hinton (1996) suggests that older cancer patients often have limited access to the full range of palliative care services. Decisions about service provision may be influenced by an ageist ideology which assumes that older people are less affected by a cancer diagnoses, more accepting of death and seem to experience less distress from symptoms. This raises an important question about ageism in practice. Many anecdotal examples indicate that younger people are perceived to have more complex problems than older people and are more likely to be admitted to a hospice in-patient unit. Palliative care services appear to have developed a culture where resources are targeted positively at younger people, for example the provision of a day service for younger people in hospice units. Healthcare services may apply age criteria at the point of delivery. This concept has been adopted by some palliative care providers and can affect access to services. Older people are viewed as having the potential to occupy in-patient beds for prolonged periods due to an acute shortage of specialist nursing home placements.

There is some evidence to indicate that patients over the age of 85 are less likely to have their palliative care needs met than younger groups. Bernabei *et al.* (1998) suggested that amongst this group of patients with chronic pain, 29 per cent reported pain daily and of these 26 per cent received no analgesia. Older people who are dying in residential and nursing homes are particularly disadvantaged. Nursing and residential home staff often fail to seek advice on pain management from palliative care professionals (Maddocks and Parker 2001).

Palliative care needs of older people

Seymour (2003) sought to provide an understanding of what was important to older people about end of life care, by exploring older peoples views, knowledge, and risk perceptions regarding the use of health technologies. Seymour said: 'Although death these days occurs most commonly at the end of a long life, until now we have known very little about what older people consider is important in achieving a dignified death – a basic human right for all'. The study participants felt they had a poor understanding of the clinical, ethical, and legal framework within which life prolonging technologies were used.

Trust, good communication, and the ability to weigh up the risks and benefits of such treatment plans were regarded as essential components in good end of life care. There was an emphasis on basic care and comfort at the end of life. Good pain control and involvement in decision making about difficult issues such as resuscitation were regarded as important. The study recommended that advanced care planning should take place as part of a process of discussion and review between clinicians, patients, and families. The involvement of older people in this research demonstrated a willingness to discuss these sensitive issues and contribute as potential users to the development of appropriate end of life care.

Palliative care teams need to respond by developing a support system for the dying person and family carers that provides physical, psychological, social, emotional, practical, and spiritual care, underpinned by an emphasis on choice, individuality, and the promotion of independence. The complexity of issues raised by patients and their families lends itself to a team approach. The focus of the multi-professional team is to improve quality of life, deliver a whole person approach, include the patient and significant other people in care planning, promote respect and choice and encourage open and sensitive communication.

In spite of the increasing prevalence of cancer with advancing age, little is documented about the psychological impact of living with cancer in the older age group in comparison with their younger counterparts. The social consequences of unmet need, the disruptions associated with prolonged treatments and the burden on caregivers is regarded as less intensive in older patients (Mor *et al.* 1994). Sociological and political analysis of disability in the literature reflects a focus on adults of working age. Arber and Ginn (1998) offer an explanation for this as the acceptance of society that illness and disability are normal consequences of ageing. Older people enter the research framework in studies that examine the burden on caregivers in mid life and the impact on economic opportunity in terms of restricting carers' access to paid employment. Therefore research makes it difficult to accurately evaluate the needs of older adults facing death.

Depression has major consequences for older people increasing their marginalization. It is the most common psychiatric illness among patients with life threatening disease (Lloyd-Williams 2003). Older people who are ill may become progressively removed from experiences which give meaning to their lives. Institutionalization in hospitals and nursing homes contributes to the process of depersonalization. Depression may be the result of a cumulative experience of loss over a lifetime and can be difficult for the patient to describe. Palliative care practitioners need to provide opportunities that allow the patient to describe their mood (Lloyd-Williams 2003). Therapeutic work may be offered by specialist workers within the multi-professional team. This should reflect the uniqueness of the individual experience. Such responses introduce human contact that can be hope enhancing and enrich life experience, reducing the sense of anxiety, loneliness, and despair.

Case Study

Jack was 82 when he was told about his limited prognosis at a palliative outpatient clinic. He was a retired teacher and had developed a passion for playing golf, a hobby shared with his wife, Alice. Jack's bone metastases from his cancer of the prostate now prevented him from playing and he described himself as in a pit and wanting to die. The family was expressing anger seeing him as giving up. A structured life review allowed Jack to explore his experience in childhood, his adult life reflecting on his many achievements, contribution to the local community and his current experience of illness. Through sensitive reflection, it allowed him to accept and feel affirmed and more hopeful about the future. Past loss and regrets concerning the death of their daughter, at birth, when Jack was at sea during the war were explored and he was able to share his experience with his wife and daughter. Jack began to engage with family life, making short term realistic plans. Most significant for all was his request to join Alice's card playing circle.

The social losses that confront older people who are facing death are fundamentally similar to other age groups. Sheldon (2003) suggests that these are concerned with community and relationships within the family. Decreased mobility may contribute to a gradual process of social withdrawal. Increased social isolation and inability to access information about services to improve quality of life can be changed by a sensitive assessment and appropriate palliative care provision. Older people often fear social death as the illness advances. Unhelpful assumptions that older people have lower expectations of life and are probably accustomed to isolation and loneliness should be challenged.

Facing death is often accompanied by frailty due to the ageing process and the older person may have difficulty maintaining roles and relationships within the family. Members of the multi-professional team need to consider the nature of the older person's role within the family and encourage adapted roles to be supported. Practical support may be offered to reduce isolation such as day care and volunteer schemes that provide support at home. Personal care may be given to help with washing, dressing, getting in and out of bed where mobility is limited by the illness. Advice and equipment provided by occupational therapists such as commodes, bed raisers, and hoists is invaluable enabling patients to be cared for at home.

Case Study

Ivy met Stewart, an American Serviceman, when she was 15 and they were married on her 17th birthday. They had 3 children, Suzy, Lindsey and Madeline, and 7 grandchildren. Recently, Ivy now aged 73, experienced a recurrence of her breast cancer with lung and cerebral metastases. She was physically frail and exhausted. Stewart was the full time carer with Lindsey helping out 2 days a week. He found it difficult to express his profound sense of loss as he struggled to cope with Ivy's increasing restlessness and anxiety. Ivy was offered an opportunity to attend the palliative care day centre. The physiotherapist worked with the day centre nurse and volunteers to build Ivy's self-confidence and improve her mobility. She appeared to become less anxious. At home, the occupational therapist introduced her to a range of equipment, including a stair lift, to promote independence. Stewart was offered counselling by a specialist social worker who talked with him about his sense of feeling overwhelmed by the loss. The professionals involved monitored and reviewed the needs of Ivy and her family on a regular basis to ensure continuity of care.

Ethnic minority elders

According to a report 'Minority Elderly Care in Europe' by the Policy Research Institute for Ageing and Ethnicity (2003), care providers are overlooking the needs of older people from a wide variety of ethnic groups, the largest being those from the Black and Asian communities. The welfare of older people in 27 minority groups across 10 countries was assessed. The report suggests that older members of ethnic minority communities would use a range of health and social care services if they were accessible, appropriate for them and adequate in terms of their social and cultural needs. For Asian communities, in particular, voluntary groups such as The Asian People with Disabilities Alliance Group (Apda) play a major part in communicating about care needs, often across a language barrier. Such groups offer older people a refuge from loneliness and isolation and a place where they can be informed of their rights.

Commenting on the Minority Elderly Care in Europe Report (Patel 2003) indicated that mainstream services are failing elder ethnic minorities. The report suggests that care providers have perpetuated a notion that these groups do not need services and this is reflected in the lack of provision. People from non-western cultures often have different concepts and beliefs about health and illness than those from the West. Ill health may be attributed to bad luck or punishment and these views may be deeply held. Alibhai-Brown (1998) suggests that the nature of care required and received by older people from ethnic minority groups is influenced by their history, memories, culture, and religion, cultural changes in mainstream and minority communities, changes in policy, law, and public attitudes towards older people in general. Continuing problems of marginalization and discrimination increase the likelihood of older people from minority ethnic communities being unable to access services such as palliative care.

Practice must be anti-discriminatory and individual beliefs and identity responded to in a culturally sensitive way. Communication must be clear and individuals' own rights and choices should be given priority. Palliative care services should be underpinned by equal opportunity policies. A locality database giving a breakdown of ethnic and religious background, age, gender, and disability should be accessible to the multi-disciplinary team. Practice could be enhanced by palliative care teams developing an active relationship with local ethnic communities.

Needs of older carers

Dying alone and unsupported can be particularly disturbing for older adults who often have an acute fear of becoming a burden on others. There are increasing numbers of seriously ill people choosing to remain at home to die (Seale and Cartwright 1994) and this brings into sharp focus the role of family caregivers. Caring for someone who is dying is a unique and personal experience. There is a complex and changing relationship between the caregiver, the ill person and other formal and informal caregivers. Some carers, particularly if they are older themselves, may be unable to access emotional and practical support to meet their specific needs and as such have the potential to be disadvantaged.

For professionals and families, it is important to clarify differences in the interpretation of role of carer (Nolan 2001). This requires openness in communication to avoid family members taking on inappropriate roles and responsibilities. Discussion about expectations can be included within the assessment and incorporated into the plan of care. This should be reviewed and adapted to reflect changes in the situation. The carer must be involved in discussions about future support and encouraged to retain control. Support may be offered through appropriate advice giving or counselling or practical assistance with personal hygiene: bathing, washing, mouth care, and attending to pressure areas. The carer may need help with moving and turning, administering medication, toileting, and incontinence problems, wound dressings and other clinical procedures. Support at night may need to be planned for and provided by specialist nursing services.

When the patient is dying the carer must be given appropriate, clear information about what to expect both before and after the death as this may be their first experience of caring for a dying person. A multi-professional team approach will help to integrate the different levels of support allowing the carer to be reassured that help will be available as new challenges arise.

Case Study

Bessie, 89, cared for her son, Samuel, who had advanced cancer of the penis and chronic schizophrenia in her one bed roomed bungalow. Bessie had a complicated history of loss in her early life. Due to mental illness, her mother was unable to care for the family and Bessie was placed in care as a young child. She was removed from a children's home by her mother 9 years later. Bessie was married at 18 and she had 2 sons, Tony and Samuel. Being a good mother was very important to Bessie and she was devoted to caring for Samuel, taking him to live with her as his care needs increased. Her husband had died 2 years previously and her beloved dog 6 months before.

Bessie was supported by a team of carers and district nurses who visited twice daily to manage Samuel's fungating wound. They helped Samuel retain his dignity and independence by taking responsibility for intimate personal care. Bessie's worries and concerns were listened to daily and her role as carer was affirmed. The specialist palliative care nurses advised on pain management. Therapeutic work was undertaken separately with Bessie who wanted to tell the story about the trauma of the separations she had experienced as a child. This loss had resurfaced as she began to think about Samuel's death. Samuel died peacefully at home in a single bed with his mother at his side.

Three months after the death Bessie said goodbye to her son, the team who had cared for them both throughout the illness, her home and community and made the journey to South Africa to continue her life with Tony her surviving son.

Physical problems, continuous nights of interrupted sleep and lack of support can lead to increased stress and tiredness. Many carers find that their health suffers because of exhaustion. Caring can also cause financial hardship due to increased laundry, heating costs, and special dietary requirements.

A survey by The Caring Costs Alliance (1996) revealed that 56 per cent of mid life carers faced future financial problems due to lost opportunities to build up savings and pensions. Isolation and loneliness are frequently experienced by carers who may spend several days and weeks alone with the dying older person. This may be intensified if the person being cared for has communication problems. With carefully planned help and support, this can be a rewarding experience for both the patient and carer. Multi-professional teams should support carers in creative ways, involving them in a process where the benefits are reciprocal, thus focusing on the more positive aspects of caring and giving meaning to the care giving relationship (Miller and Powell-Lawton 1997).

Where do older people die?

One of the most difficult dilemmas for an older person who is seriously ill is about where they are going to be cared for when they are dying. Older people need to be given appropriate information about residential and nursing homes, hospice inpatient, and care at home to enable them to make an informed choice about their end of life care. In reality, many older people have a limited choice and move into residential care because they are unable to be supported at home. Sheldon (2003), reports that age, gender, and social class are factors that are likely to influence the decision to move into a supervised care situation. Older women who have survived their spouse and are living in poverty are more likely to end their lives in care.

Case Study

Sylvia, aged 78, had moved from Hungary with her husband Mickel in 1956. They had one daughter, Maria, who had moved to Australia six years ago. Mickel died eighteen months later. Sylvia said that this was due to a broken heart. Her cancer of the ovary was diagnosed four months after Mickel's death. During the past year Maria had spent extended periods in England caring for her mother.

Sylvia's condition deteriorated after Maria returned to Australia and she was admitted to the hospice. Following a period of respite care in the hospice ward, options for Sylvia's future care were considered. The transition was supported by a plan to give appropriate information about the choices available. The Care Manager acted as the key worker and communicated with Maria by email. Sylvia was kept informed and involved in all discussions about her future, maximizing control and choice. The multi-professional team ensured that the transition to the nursing home was timed appropriately. The care staff at the home were familiar with Sylvia's needs before her discharge from the hospice. The future level of support to be provided by the specialist palliative care team was defined and agreed. Sylvia died peacefully seven weeks later in the nursing home of her choice.

Entering care can be a challenging experience, for the older person and the family members. The change may be accompanied by feelings of guilt as the family adapt to the new situation that may require them to meet financial commitments towards the cost of care. These changes represent losses in themselves and may complicate the adjustment to bereavement. There are recognized areas for development if dying is to be managed well in nursing homes: funding constraints, public perception of low standards of care, and the culture of care that exists where the emphasis is on living and dying people are marginalized (Field and Frogatt 2003).

The majority of people who die in nursing homes do so from some chronic disabling condition other than cancer. There would appear to be a culture of care in some of these institutions that fails to promote an acceptance of dying. Training programmes should be developed and delivered by palliative care teams to raise awareness and inform care home staff about good practice in end of life care. Communication systems must be set up between palliative care services and nursing homes to ensure that specialist advice and support continues throughout the illness experience. There should be a seamless transition if the move is from a hospice inpatient unit to a nursing home. Admission to nursing and residential homes should not imply reduced access to palliative care services. Some hospices increase the marginalization of older people who have entered care by including criteria which exclude older people in care from access to palliative day care.

With an increasing numbers of seriously ill people remaining at home to die, consideration must be given to carers needs in palliative care provision. Higginson (2003) reports that 49 per cent of people over 65 indicate that they would choose to be cared for at home. Inpatient hospice care represents second choice with 23 per cent. Given effective planning and partnership working, a range of services can be provided to enable the older person to remain at home. In fact, most people spend 90 per cent of the last year of life in their own homes (Grande and Addington-Hall 1998).

A patient and family centred approach to decision making about future care avoids options being discussed arbitrarily with the individual in isolation. Pressures about bed blocking in hospitals and hospice inpatient units may obscure this process. Interventions that enable the older person to find a new role within the family and remain included can be empowering.

Case Study

Stephan, who had advanced cancer of the lung, lived alone supported by his daughter Shirley and her partner. Stephan was housebound and dependent on his daughter to provide personal care. Stephan was feeling worthless and Shirley became increasingly exhausted with the demands of his care. Following a joint assessment including Stephan and Shirley, by the occupational therapist, social worker, specialist palliative care nurse and care manager, it was agreed that Stephan would move to Shirley's home for weekends. It would then be possible to be involved more actively in family life. For a short time, he was able to advise on the rebuilding of a car engine project being undertaken by his grandson. Other family members reconnected with Stephan and offered to relieve Shirley of the care two days a week. Shirley had a course of reflexology at the hospice and one week of respite care was agreed for a future date.

Palliative care workers have a role in facilitating this process; dealing with change, conflict and loss, maximizing strengths, and identifying coping strategies within the whole family. A collaborative approach between the older person, the family, and all the stakeholders involved is likely to produce the most effective result.

Bereavement care

Older people are as vulnerable as any other age group when bereavement occurs. Assumptions may be made that due to the cumulative loss experience throughout life, older people are less affected by death than other age groups. There are many examples in practice where older people have experienced multiple losses that have complicated the bereavement. Some argue that older people have been exposed to a culture where emotional expression was minimized and therefore to offer a therapeutic response which involves expression of grief is inappropriate. Scrutton (1995) challenges such ageist ideas that produce a social climate that promotes a negative view of older people and may have an impact on whether or not they receive appropriate bereavement care. The pain of separation and loss with its social and emotional consequences is unaffected by age.

Decisions about what support to offer in bereavement need to be considered alongside consideration of psychological and emotional strength and resilience. There may be an attempt to minimize the impact of the loss, its significance, and the genuineness of the grief. Older people need to be given the choice to decide what bereavement support is appropriate.

The uniqueness of grief reactions needs to be the focus of our under-standing. While there may be evidence of distress, some older people may choose not to display an emotional response and may internalize their reaction. Therapeutic interventions should involve flexibility, creativity, and recognize the individuality of each bereavement experience. Older people need to have their experience of bereavement validated and under-stood within the context of early attachment. Early losses such as stillbirths may be brought into focus as the older person experiences the losses asso-ciated with dying. Support should be offered that affirms memories and maximizes individual coping strategies.

Conclusion

Robinson (2002) reported that assumptions about old age being a time of inevitable ill health and dwindling personal capacity pervades health and social care and in fact much of society. Older people state repeatedly that they wish to live independently with dignity and equal access to health and social care. Public services across the country are failing to meet even the most basic needs. Robinson suggests that the solutions to ageism in health and social care include the introduction of legislation to prevent unfair discrimination, an increase in spending on older people's services, better training and support for care workers, and the involvement of older people in service planning. Palliative care services need to provide flexible and equitable care, responsive to need, underpinned by sensitive communica-tion, and a creativity that demonstrates appreciation of the uniqueness of each individual experience regardless of chronological age.

References

Alibhai-Brown Y (1998) *Caring for Ethnic Minority Elders: A Guide*. Age Concern, London.

Arber S and Ginn J (1998) Health and illness in later life. In Field D and Taylor S (ed.) *Sociological Perspectives on Health and Illness*. Blackwell Scientific.

Asian People with Disabilities Alliance web site at: http://www.apda.org.uk.

Bernabei R, Gambassi G, and Lapane K (1998) The management of chronic pain in older persons. *Journal of American Geriatric Society* 46:635–51.

Butler RN (1969). Ageism: another form of bigotry. *The Gerontologist* 9:243–6.

Centre for Policy on Ageing (1996) *A Better Home Life*. Centre for Policy on Ageing, London.

Department of Health (2000) The NHS cancer plan. A plan for investment. A plan for reform. Department of Health, London.

Department of Health (2001a) Care homes for older people. National minimum standards. The Stationery Office, London.

Department of Health (2001b) National service framework for older people. Department of Health, London.

Department for Works & Pensions (2001) Income related benefits – estimates of take up in 1999/2000, DWP, tables 1.1, 2.1 and 3.1.

Field D and Froggatt K (2003) Issues for palliative care in nursing and residential homes. In Katz JS and Peace S (ed.) *End of Life in Care Homes.* Oxford University Press, Oxford.

Living in Britain: results from the 2000 General Household Survey (GHS), ONS, Crown Copyright 2001, table 7.1 (Trends in self-reported sickness by age and sex).

Grande G and Addington-Hall J (1998) Place of death and access to home care: are certain groups at a disadvantage? *Social Science Medicine* 47:565–79.

Higginson I (2003) Priorities and preferences for end of life care in England, Scotland and Wales. National Council for Hospice and Specialist Palliative Care Services, London.

Hinton J (1996) Services given and help perceived during home care for terminal cancer. *Palliative Medicine* 10:125–34.

Lloyd-Williams M (2003) Screening for depression in palliative care. In Lloyd-Williams M (ed.) *Psychosocial Issues in Palliative Care.* Oxford University Press, Oxford.

Maddocks I and Parker D (2001) Palliative care in nursing homes. In Addington-Hall J and Higginson I (ed.) *Palliative Care for Non-Cancer Patients*, pp. 147–57. Oxford University Press, Oxford.

Miller B and Powell-Lawton M (1997) Symposium – positive aspects of caregiving: finding balance in caregiving research. *Gerontologist* 37(2):216–7.

Mor V, Allen S, and Malin M (1994) The psychosocial impact of cancer on older versus younger patients and their families. *Cancer Supplement*, October 7, 1994, 74(7).

NICE (2003) Supportive and palliative care cancer service guidance (Draft). National Institute for Clinical Excellence, London.

Nolan M (2001) Positive aspects of caring. In Payne S and Ellis-Hill C (ed.) *Chronic and Terminal Illness New Perspectives on Caring and Carers.* Oxford University Press, Oxford.

Patel N (ed.) (2003) Minority elderly care in Europe. Report by the policy research institute for ageing and ethnicity.

Peace S (2003) The development of residential and nursing home care in the United Kingdom. In Katz JS and Peace S (ed.) *End of Life in Care Homes. A Palliative Care Approach*, pp.15–42. Oxford University Press. Oxford.

Robinson J (2002) Old habits die hard. *Tackling Age Discrimination in Health and Social Care*. The Kings Fund, London.

Scrutton S (1995) *Bereavement and Grief, Supporting Older People Through Loss*. Age Concern England, London.

Seale C and Cartright A (1994) *The Year Before Death*. Aldershot, Avesbury.

Seymour J (2003) Technology and Natural Death: a study of older people. Web site at: *http://www.shef.ac.uk/uni/projects/gop/index.htm*

Sheldon F (2003) Social impact of advanced metastatic cancer. In Lloyd-Williams M (ed.) *Psychosocial Issues in Palliative Care*. Oxford University Press, Oxford.

Statistics from Age Concern web site at: *http://www.ageconcern.org.uk/acherts/info_339.htm*

Statistics from Alzheimer's Society web site at: *http://www.alzheimers.org.uk/about/statistics/html.*

General Social Care Council Codes of Conduct (2003) General Social Care Council web site at: *http://www.gscc.org.uk*

The Caring Costs Alliance (1996) The true costs of caring: a survey of carers lost income. London.

Townsend P (1962) *The Last Refuge*. Routledge and Kegan, London.

6

Mental health needs

Max Henderson

Exclusion of individuals with mental health problems from social roles and opportunities preceded the identification of their difficulties as 'mental health' in origin. Ideas of possession or 'animality', in which the madman was 'not sick' but in fact 'protected ... from whatever might be fragile, precarious or sickly in man', underlay 'treatment' with forced labour or confinement in the eighteenth century (Foucault 1965). It is striking that as lunacy has been reconstructed as illness, its management brought within the professional bounds of medicine, and effective biological treatments developed, nonetheless views of deviance and 'otherness' remain.

This chapter will examine the way in which those with long-term mental health problems are voiceless; such voicelessness is to a degree entwined with the nature of their illness. This limited ability to make their needs known contributes substantially to their ongoing suffering. The interaction of mental health difficulties with palliative medicine merits close attention. This should help identify opportunities to restructure the relationship and thereby give this group a greater voice and better care.

Long-term mental health problems

There is a growing awareness of the prevalence of mental illness within society. This includes the highest sanction of mental health being identified by the government as one of its top three health priorities (Department of Health 2002). Some mental illnesses are more of a problem than others. How much of a problem depends on whom is being asked. Economically, depression is the greatest mental health problem (UNUM 2001). The number of days lost from work and the cost of prescriptions for antidepressant drugs places a substantial burden on the nation's finances. However, most people get better from depression. Anxiety disorders, both discretely and in the context of depression, contribute to individual social disability. Abuse of alcohol and other substances is increasing, yet the uneasy way this sits with what is or is not socially acceptable means its impact on individuals and society remains largely unknown.

The burden of the psychotic disorders, principally schizophrenia, is much more clear. The destruction of personality, relationships, and social roles is easily demonstrated, together with the fact that schizophrenia usually persists as a chronic disorder, despite some striking improvements in its symptomatic management. Schizophrenia typically develops in the second and third decade and often progresses to a chronic syndrome. The features of the acute syndrome include delusions, where an individual holds usually false beliefs which are unusual in terms of that person's background and are held on inadequate grounds; hallucinations where the individual experiences perceptions in the absence of external stimuli; and disorders of thinking where, for example, the individual will allude to an experience of thoughts which he knows not to be his, or where he perceives his thoughts to be accessible to others without his control. Current anti-psychotic medication is effective at alleviating these symptoms, though relapses can occur at times of stress or if compliance with medication is poor. The chronic syndrome of schizophrenia, which has proved much less amenable to treatment, is characterized by 'negative' symptoms. These include apathy, emotional blunting, and social withdrawal in the context of limited or absent insight. Additional depressive features occur in about one-third of patients. The lifetime risk of schizophrenia is approximately 1%, although there is recent evidence of an increased risk within the UK Afro-Caribbean population, the causes of which have yet to be fully elucidated (Boydell *et al.* 2001).

Another group of conditions, also associated with substantial changes in personality, are the dementias. These are acquired conditions in which there is generalized and progressive impairment of intellect, memory, and personality. That these occur within clear consciousness distinguishes them from delirium. Loss of memory is often the presenting feature of dementia, but in time changes in thinking and behaviour occur. Depression, hallucinations, and delusions can also be part of the clinical picture. The most common cause of dementia in the UK remains Alzheimer's disease but there is increasing recognition of cerebro-vascular disease and dementia with Lewy bodies (Ritchie and Lovestone 2002). The prevalence of Alzheimer's disease increases with increasing age. Less than 5% of those aged under 65 are affected but by 80, 1 in 5 are sufferers. The total number of individuals with dementia is increasing as the population gets older. Treatments have been developed that can stabilize or even improve the cognitive decline experienced by these patients. The effects are, however, small and do not represent a cure.

Mental health in palliative care

Emotional and psychological care has been important for palliative care since its inception. There have been two broad areas involved, that of the patient and that of the bereaved relative. The study of bereavement, and in particular pathological bereavement reactions has developed an independence and structure of its own (Parkes 1972). Research into psychiatric problems experienced by palliative care patients has developed less quickly. Possible reasons for this include the belief that symptoms such as depression and anxiety are either normal or untreatable in this population (Massie 1989). Such nihilism of course stands in marked contrast to the substantial improvements that are known to be available for 'physical' symptoms such as pain and nausea. Palliative care doctors are still poor at both recognizing and treating depression in a palliative care setting (Fallowfield *et al.* 2001). The body of research on the subject is both small and of variable quality. Nevertheless improvements are taking place, with interest both in the UK and North America. An example of this has been the publication of the first major textbook in the field (Chochinov and Breitbart 2000). Even in a dedicated book, the chapter on palliative care needs of those with long-term mental health problems is amongst the briefest. This is not to say it has been ignored by the editors but rather that the thinking and published work upon which they could draw is so limited. In this situation we must look more widely, into broader psycho-oncology, psychiatry itself, and groups with potentially similar difficulties such as learning difficulties (see Chapter 7) for evidence to guide us.

General health care for those with long-term mental health problems

Patients with long-term mental health problems are also users of 'physical' health services. Any journey that encompasses time engaged with palliative medicine will have started with care from primary and, almost certainly, secondary care. Before any attempt is made to examine the interface between chronic mental ill health and palliative care, events that occur earlier (in primary and secondary care) but which may bias events when the palliative stage is reached, should be studied.

The separation of physical medicine and psychiatric medicine physically, professionally and, at times, philosophically, produces difficulties for those areas at their interface. In particular this includes patients with unexplained physical symptoms, unloved by physicians and surgeons (Anonymous 1978), or patients with both medical and psychological pathologies. These groups are poorly served by health services as currently configured (Felker *et al.* 1996; Karasu *et al.* 1980).

A relevant area where mental health patients seem disadvantaged is that of screening for cancer. In a recent study by Wernecke and colleagues, the uptake of breast and cervical screening by patients receiving care in a psychiatric hospital was audited (Werneke *et al.* in press). Those women with severe mental illness, mainly schizophrenia and bipolar disorder, were significantly less likely to attend breast screening (odds ratio 0.50, 95% CI 0.36–0.69) or cervical screening (odds ratio 0.80, 95% CI 0.68–0.94). In women who had abnormal colposcopy results, significantly fewer of those with mental health problems returned for proper assessment.

Normally, for symptoms to attract medical attention, patients need to 'complain'. Although this sounds obvious, that only serves to underline that this simple step is taken for granted. The individual needs to perceive a bodily sensation as concerning, conclude that it requires medical attention and explain this to a doctor. Each of these parts is in turn made up of smaller decisions and actions. A number of core difficulties of a patient with chronic schizophrenia could prevent some of these actions taking place. A suspicious patient, already suffering with unpleasant auditory hallucinations or a belief that another person has control over his thoughts or his bodily functions may not recognize a new physical perception as sinister or requiring medical attention (Talbott and Linn 1978). The pervasive apathy of the negative syndrome of schizophrenia might prevent that patient seeking medical attention even if he believes it necessary. The difficulties with processing thoughts that interfere with effective communication might prevent the patient accurately describing his symptoms in a way that a doctor would recognize as deserving of further attention.

Physical complaints in patients with known psychiatric disorder can be ascribed to their underlying mental illness, and not given sufficient credence (Henderson 2000). Evidence suggests that physicians find psychiatric patients unrewarding (Ansel and McGee 1971; Patel 1975; Ramon and Breyter 1978; Karasu *et al.* 1980). Their behavioural problems can make them unwelcome in clinic settings (Garai and Goldsmith 1979; Karasu *et al.* 1980). Their difficulties in adhering to management plans can infuriate (McConnell *et al.* 1992). The sharp division that exists between physical and psychological medicine frequently means that a practitioner in one lacks skills or confidence in examining the other. Liaison psychiatrists have demonstrated that hospital doctors miss psychiatric illness in their patients (Maguire *et al.* 1974; Mayou and Hawton 1986; Feldman *et al.* 1987; Balestrieri *et al.* 2002), but there is also evidence that psychiatrists are reluctant to physically examine their patients (McIntyre and Romano 1977).

This inequity is more concerning given that the presence of a psychiatric illness has implications in terms of morbidity and mortality (Hoenig and Hamilton 1966; Koranyi 1979; Maricle *et al.* 1987*a, b*). Those with chronic mental illness typically lead less healthy lives. They indulge in more unhealthy activities such as smoking, drinking, and poor diets (Koranyi 1979). They take less exercise.

Palliative care for patients with mental health problems

Whilst both psychosis and dementia might both handicap a patient in accessing general health care, they raise different questions in terms of access to palliative care. The challenges faced by patients and carers when a patient with a chronic psychotic illness also has a terminal illness will be addressed in due course. These might be seen as distinct from the problems of the demented patient as one might argue that dementia itself is a condition requiring palliative care.

Dementia

Dementia is typically a disease of old age. Diagnosis is most common in the 70s and the approximate time to death is 10 years. This figure is however variable for two reasons. Firstly the time-course and natural history of the disease is still not fully known and is therefore difficult to predict. Secondly in the eighth and ninth decades patients are vulnerable to a number of diseases and in fact most dementia patients die of another illness such as diabetes or coronary heart disease. However in many patients there is a recognizable end stage lasting 2–3 years (Shuster, Jr. 2000). This is characterized by a wide range of symptoms which have in common that they are progressive, irreversible, and often destructive to the integrity of the patient as an individual (Table 6.1).

There would seem to be little doubt that the broad symptom complex of end stage dementia would benefit from a palliative care approach (Marsh *et al.* 2000; Shuster, Jr. 2000). In particular the carers of these patients have

Table 6.1 Features of Advanced Dementia

Neurocognitive	Worsening memory
	Confusion/disorientation
	Irritability
	Apathy
Psychiatric	Hallucinations
	Delusions
	Depression
Physical	Poor swallowing → risk of aspiration
	Loss of mobility
	Incontinence
	Pain
Social	Loss of roles
	Relationship changes
	Concerns about separation, abandonment, dying
Complications	Skin damage
	Urinary infections
	Chest infections

much to gain. Yet this group are still largely excluded from palliative care support. Hanrahan and Luchins in a survey of American hospices found that only 21% were admitting patients with dementia (Hanrahan and Luchins 1995). As a result less than 1% of the 250,000 US hospice patients had a primary diagnosis of dementia. It is likely that a similar situation pertains in the UK. Little is known about how and where the needs of end stage dementia patients are being met. For such patients to be cared for at home their carers must feel able to provide a sufficient level of care. There is a certain irony in the fact that the very length of the illness may leave the carer exhausted and feeling unable to continue. The result is often that patients are admitted into institutional care such as a nursing home. Whilst there are many examples of excellent care in such settings, few would claim to offer true palliative care.

Why is it that end stage dementia patients are not receiving the palliative care their symptoms suggest they should? One reason is the difficulty in predicting the time to death in demented patients; 80% of the hospices in the survey by Hanrahan and Luchins report this as their major difficulty. Modern palliative medicine has evolved from a much narrower focus on terminal care; that is, care just shortly before death where the time to death is predictable (Saunders 2001). Such an evolution is welcome in the face of technological and medical advances which have led to the prolongation of the 'terminal' phase of many illnesses. However, the discomfort felt by palliative medicine in dealing with patients whose prognosis is relatively long or uncertain continues. In the UK where access to palliative care is via the normal NHS system (even though much of its funding comes from charitable sources) there are no hard rules about life expectancy. Patients with longer life expectancies are sometimes treated in palliative care units but efforts are made to discharge them back to primary care when the goals of the referral have been met. Such a discharge would be difficult to effect in the case of dementia. In the United States where access is regulated by patients' medical insurance policy, fees will not be met if the patient has more than six months to live. The ability of physicians to predict this is limited (Volicer *et al.* 1993). Several tools to predict when the dementia patient has less than six months to live have been studied (Reisberg 1988; Marsh *et al.* 2000). Such research of course is of little intrinsic use to the patient and one could argue that it might be self-fulfilling. Nothing in the published literature tells us what happens to those whose level of need would permit them access to palliative care but whose life expectancy is too great.

Presumably those with less than six months *do* access this care? Christakas and Escarce have found that the median survival time of dementia patients after a hospice admission is 36 days (Christakis and Escarce 1996). This suggests that these patients are accessing care only in the very last stages.

There are other reasons why traditional palliative medicine might be reluctant to make itself available to dementia patients. Communication lies at the heart of good palliative care which emerged at a time when discussions about death and terminal illness were not only taboo but felt to be harmful to the patient. Part of its holistic approach was to create a safe environment where patients and professionals could discuss such issues with the aim of maximizing the patients' control, and hence dignity, in their final phase of life. Doctors and nurses in the specialty are justifiably proud of their communication skills. But what if the patient cannot communicate or express their needs? The process of palliation might be hampered at a very early stage. The professional is less able to use their listening and empathic skills to make the patient feel secure. They are less able to use their diagnostic skills to formulate the cause of the patient's complaint. As a result they will find alleviating such symptoms, by both pharmacological and non-pharmacological means, very difficult. Additionally, and not to be underestimated, they are unlikely to receive feedback suggesting that the efforts have been successful.

It has been suggested that demented patients have a higher pain threshold than non-demented patients but evidence for this is weak (Farrell *et al.* 1996; Donovan 1997). Pain is under-treated in dementia (Farrell *et al.* 1996; Weissman and Matson 1999). Healthcare professionals including those in palliative care often see a strong correlation between pain behaviour and level of suffering. Leaving aside discussion of how strong this correlation is in the traditional palliative care population, it is weak in cognitively impaired populations. The cognitive model of pain divides pain into four psychological dimensions—pain sensation, pain evaluation, pain affect, and pain behaviour (Turk and Okifuji 2002). Differences in pain sensation are unlikely and would be difficult to demonstrate. Conversely, that dementia patients might evaluate their subjective experience of pain differently seems entirely plausible. Such evaluation requires the experience to be set in the context of both the present environment and past experience. Aspects of cognitive impairment will make one or both difficult. Pain behaviour in dementia patients can be atypical, such as grimacing or posturing (Shuster, Jr. 2000). Alternatively the behaviour might be normal but the intensity may be unusual, such that objectively greater stimuli produce a muted response and minor stimuli produce an exaggerated response. All behaviours will, as in the non-demented population, be modified by the patients' mood state—another difficult area to assess in cognitively impaired patients. Manfredi videotaped the facial expressions of dementia patients before and during a dressing change (Manfredi *et al.* 2003). The tapes were then randomized and shown to assessors blind to whether or not the patients were having the procedure. There was significant agreement between the assessors as to whether or not the patient was in pain although they were not able to agree about the *intensity* of this pain. Lane and colleagues have included assessment of facial expression into their PAINAD scale for the assessment of pain in dementia (Lane *et al.* 2003). Here assessments of five potential markers of pain are scored in a 0/1/2 basis, giving a score out of 10. Further studies using the scale are awaited. Nonetheless its existence highlights the need to find innovative ways to assess symptoms in patients who are unable to express themselves adequately.

Schizophrenia

In contrast to most cases of dementia, the onset of schizophrenia is in young adult life. It typically follows a chronic course. The palliative care literature has not focused on the end of life needs of patients who develop a life-threatening illness on a background of schizophrenia although the National Council for Hospice and Specialist Palliative Care Services has produced an 'Occasional Paper' on the subject (Addington-Hall J 2000). Within the peer-reviewed literature there is a single case report of the hospice care delivered to a schizophrenic patient which concludes that 'the area merits further description and investigation' (Kelly and Shanley 2000) and an editorial written by both a palliative care specialist and two psychiatrists that details how each area of medicine can influence and educate the other (Spiess *et al.* 2002).

At least two aspects of the possible management of chronic schizophrenic patients merit attention. The first is the difficult social milieu in which such patients often find themselves and the second is the thorny area of stigma. Palliative care places emphasis on holistic care of the patient. An important aspect of this is the social and family environment in which the patient exists. Efforts are made to engage with the patients family, to explain what treatment options exist and ultimately to support the family through bereavement. Families and carers are a vital part of the process and can be utilized for example to collect, administer or simply encourage adherence to medication, or for a corroborating account of changes in symptoms. The sometimes parlous social situation of the chronic schizophrenic patient is so much more (and less) than just the absence of a carer. Social withdrawal is a core feature of the negative syndrome of schizophrenia. Contact with others is avoided. Social interests can be minimal and interactions awkward and uncomfortable for both parties. The 'positive' syndrome can be socially unattractive also, with disinhibited or odd behaviours, restlessness or irritability. Many chronic schizophrenic patients will have worked at best infrequently and never had financial independence from the benefits system. For both medical and economic reasons many live in hostels with variable levels of support. The contrast between the warm family environment of some palliative care patients and that of the chronic schizophrenic can be marked. The physical surroundings of a hostel might be threatening and the lack of a supportive carer to assist with activities of daily living or medication frustrating almost as much for the palliative care worker as for the patient. The nature of the negative syndrome means patients will often not present the same warm persona that many of even the sickest patients do. It is easy to see that unconsciously, and despite high levels of professionalism, engagement with such difficult patients can be less deep than with more straightforward patients.

That psychiatric patients are stigmatized is beyond doubt (Hayward and Bright 1997). Stigma refers to the negative effects of a label placed on a group. Many studies describe the negative ways in which individuals with mental illness are viewed by society. One early study found that the public thought that psychiatric patients were 'dirty, unintelligent, insincere, and worthless' (Nunnally 1961). Hayward and Bright have attempted to distil the root causes of such stigmatizing attitudes into four factors: dangerousness, attribution of responsibility, poor prognosis, and disruption of social interactions. Might any of these apply to palliative care professionals and institutions?

There is nothing in the literature to inform us about dangerousness in palliative care, although perhaps now more than ever the general public do perceive severe mental illness as intrinsically related to a high risk of violence though psychiatric patients contribute a very small proportion of the violent acts committed. The idea of attribution of responsibility is that somehow psychiatric patients 'choose' to become mentally ill. One way of understanding this view of the mentally ill is as a self-protection device. People who conclude that patients are responsible for their predicament can come to the comfortable conclusion that they themselves will not become ill in this way (Lerner and Miller 1978).

The possibility that professionals in palliative care might find psychiatric patients unrewarding to treat has already been alluded to. Whilst there is no evidence from studies in palliative care itself, the attitudes of both medical students and hospital doctors to psychiatric patients has been studied. In one survey half the sample of medical students agreed with the statement: 'psychiatric patients generally speaking are not easy to like' (Wilkinson et al. 1983). This proportion increased when the subjects were re-surveyed two years post-qualification (Sivakumar et al. 1986). More senior hospital doctors, who have presumably been more exposed to psychiatric patients than their junior colleagues, have less negative attitudes to psychiatric patients (Patel 1975). Exposure to psychiatric patients does seem to ameliorate attitudes (Whately 1959), though in this respect the small number of such patients receiving palliative care suggests that current attitudes will remain in place.

The final explanation for stigmatizing attitudes is that the mentally ill do not fit into normal patterns of social interaction *and people do not feel comfortable in situations where the normal rules of social interaction do not function.* Much of this social role disruption model was initially described by Goffman (Goffman 1968). Palliative care is a highly social activity, with the development of close relationships between patient and professional at a difficult time in life. There is intimate contact—patients may be in bed, less than fully clothed, or in their private homes. Very private personal feelings and beliefs are discussed in a way which does not happen in everyday social intercourse. Even the slightest preconceived idea that in embarking on such social contact, one might get an unpredictable or awkward response will to some degree influence how one initiates contact.

Learning lessons

When palliative care began, at least in its modern form, some forty years ago, it needed to define itself and make clear how it was different. It did so by making a firm boundary between itself and other forms of medicine and social care. This was crucial in enabling a discrete identity to develop. In time it has expanded with the shift from terminal care to a broader focus on end of life issues. However, this has been a relatively small change—most palliative care patients have cancer and most are in the last few months of life. There have been some developments with increasing interest in the palliative care of diseases such as motor neurone disease, AIDS and congestive cardiac failure though these still account for a small fraction of the overall palliative care population.

Whilst palliative care's view of itself has remained focussed on retaining its boundaries, its place within medicine has changed: it is now mainstream. Most large hospitals have access to at least some palliative care, and there are substantive academic posts and several learned journals dedicated to researching the field. Even the UK's new 'Cancer Czar' is a palliative care physician. That this is so should be greeted warmly by the specialty. Saunders and those who have followed her have correctly recognized an area of medical care poorly provided for by other specialties and, moreover, have successfully begun to address the problem. However, with this burgeoning maturity come new responsibilities. No longer can palliative care focus on a narrow exclusive field. An examination of the attitudes of palliative care to patients with long-term mental health problems can not only help to illuminate this modern tension within palliative care but also perhaps assist in finding solutions.

There is almost no literature on the palliative care needs of patients with severe mental illnesses such as schizophrenia. In this respect palliative care is not unique—this just reflects the wider difficulties that psychiatric patients have in obtaining equitable medical care. It is however an issue that palliative care should address. This should first be done by examining how palliative care is delivered. Are there ways in which current palliative care *structurally* excludes those with severe mental illness? Although palliative care cannot *per se* assist psychiatric patients to get physically examined by their doctors, be screened or receive active treatment for disease, they can make sure that when advanced and terminal illness comes these patients can receive the level of care their overall symptom burden demands.

There is no disputing that some patients with severe psychotic illnesses can present problems to those trying to care for them. However, this is certainly not the case for all patients, and rarely all the time for most patients. The majority of patients with long-term mental health problems will pose no problems during a palliative care admission. It is possible that some difficulties may preclude admission to units such as modern hospices—in such situations palliative care must recognize that the level of patient need still exists, indeed it is probably amplified. In addition, the staff who are caring for the patient will also have needs. The American Psychiatric Association has started to recognize these difficulties and has included a training period in palliative medicine for those wishing to undergo training in the psychiatry of old age (APA Council Resolution 2001). Perhaps palliative care could include a period of psychiatric training into its programmes? But more imaginative ways need to be found too. Whilst the chronic schizophrenic may be socially isolated he may have a long-term relationship with a key worker from a Community Mental Health Team. Could this person be treated as the patient's 'family' in terms of discussions about care? Palliative care nurses visit patients at home and talk frankly with their families—could they develop in-reach programmes to psychiatric units so that the process of palliative care for psychiatric staff can be de-mystified, and palliative care can learn from them some of the skills needed to care effectively for the chronically mentally ill? All the evidence suggests that as social distance from the mentally ill is reduced so are stigmatizing attitudes.

The difficulties in predicting time to death are real, and the possibility of scarce palliative care resources being swallowed up by the increasing numbers of dementia patients that current demographic trends predict is also real. But is this the only reason that palliative care is reluctant to respond to non-cancer dementia patients? Again the very *social* nature of palliative care is challenged by patients with limited or no ability to effectively describe or discuss their difficulties. Attempts at overcoming the difficulties that dementia patients present have started. Pain assessment tools are an example. More research is needed into the assessment and management of mood and behavioural disturbance. Methods of evaluating palliative interventions in a population unable to verbalize a response would be of great value. The protracted nature of the illness means that the bereavement experience of the families and carers of dementia patients is often difficult. As the ability to communicate with, and in many cases even recognize, family members is eroded the nature of the relationship changes. Many relatives will describe having said, 'Goodbye' long before the patient's death. What impact this will have on care-giving until death will vary with individual cases, but ambivalence and even resentment would be understandable in such situations. Palliative care has skills in bereavement issues. By the time a dementia patient is admitted, six months prior to death at best but more likely one month as things currently stand, the change to the relationship between patient and carer may have already occurred. As with psychotic patients whose behaviour may make them difficult to manage within a small hospice, wholesale absorption of all dementia patients need not occur. But palliative care must recognize that its skills are needed and appropriate for a wider patient population. Links need to be made with geriatric medicine and neurology to assist them in the appropriate management of advanced dementia patients and their families. The role of the nursing home needs close attention too. Placement in these institutions is a final common pathway for a number of challenging clinical conditions including advanced dementia and advanced Parkinson's disease where the patient's family can no longer adequately care for them at home. To what extent, and measured by which tools, such placements provide optimum care as opposed to basic safe care is worthy of examination. In-reaching of palliative care or provision of education to nursing homes with complex non-cancer residents could represent a significant advance in the care of the most difficult (and therefore often the most vulnerable) of patients.

It should not be assumed that the transfer of skills are described is a one-way process. Palliative care is and will remain a social activity inasmuch as its cornerstone is the social interactions between patient, professional, and carer. Social skills are never so good that they cannot be improved upon. The sometimes uncomfortable and challenging experience of making a detailed assessment of someone with chronic psychosis or marked cognitive impairment can be a learning experience in itself. Lessons learned from communicating with a more diverse patient population will be applicable to the patient population already well served in palliative care. Palliative care has firmly established itself as a necessary and vital part of medicine. The care of those with mental health problems presents one challenge which will need to be met if past progress is to be maintained.

Case Study

Miss W was in her 60s when she was diagnosed with myeloma. She had had a long history of a manic depression. She had spent long periods in psychiatric hospital, particularly in her younger years, but became better engaged in her later years. Her breakdowns were rare but characterized by confusion and paranoid ideas, often with over-energetic antisocial behaviour.

The haematology team and the hospital palliative care team were keen for the hospice to become involved with Miss W. However she was quite reluctant given her previous experience of what she felt was institutional care. Nonetheless her overriding wish was not to die in a psychiatric ward. The hospice whilst recognizing the appropriateness of the referral, were concerned about the possibility of her becoming psychiatrically ill whilst in the hospice, in particular there were concerns about monitoring psychiatric medication (e.g. lithium) and distinguishing 'medical' delirium from 'psychiatric' psychosis.

The availability of a liaison psychiatrist able to act as a link between the various specialties facilitated solutions to these difficulties. He was able to meet Miss W in a joint clinic appointment with her psychiatrist, being able to reassure her that her psychiatric needs could be met in the hospice. Teaching and informal support of the hospice nurse specialists allowed them to develop a close supportive arrangement with Miss W whilst she was an outpatient. This also enabled them both to identify the appropriate time for an admission for terminal care, each being confident that the multidisciplinary team could cope with any difficulties. Miss W died peacefully in the hospice, and not, as she feared, in a psychiatric ward.

Key Points

◆ Miss W reassured by presence of a psychiatrist *who was familiar with the hospice and palliative care*

◆ Psychiatrist able to educate and support hospice staff in the care of a *potentially* difficult patient

◆ **Good communication** between community psychiatry, palliative care, and hospice psychiatrist was crucial in providing individually appropriate care for a vulnerable patient

References

Addington-Hall J 2000, *Positive Partnerships. Palliative care for adults with severe mental health problems*, National Council for Hospice and Specialist Palliative Care Services and Scottish Partnership Agency for Palliative and Cancer Care, London, Occasional Paper 17.

Anonymous (1978) Taking care of the hateful patient. *N. Engl. J. Med.* **299**(7):366–7.

Ansel E and McGee R (1971) Attitudes towards suicide attempters. *Bulletin of Suicidology* **8**:22–8.

APA Council Resolution (2001) *End of Life Issues and Care for Adults.* American Psychological Association, Washington.

Balestrieri M, Bisoffi G, Tansella M, Martucci M, and Goldberg DP (2002) Identification of depression by medical and surgical general hospital physicians. *Gen. Hosp. Psychiatry* **24**(1):4–11.

Boydell J, van Os J, Mckenzie K, Allardyce J, Goel R, McCreadie RG, *et al.* (2001) Incidence of schizophrenia in ethnic minorities in London: ecological study into interactions with environment. *British Medical Journal* **323**:1336–8.

Chochinov HM and Breitbart W (2000) *Handbook of Psychiatry in Palliative Medicine.* Oxford University Press, New York.

Christakis NA and Escarce JJ (1996) Survival of medicare patients after enrollment in hospice programs. *N. Engl. J. Med.* **335**(3):172–8.

Department of Health (2002) *Saving Lives: Our Healthier Nation.* Department of Health, London.

Donovan J (1997) Learning disabilities. Pain signals. *Nurs. Times* **93**(45):60–2.

Fallowfield L, Ratcliffe D, Jenkins V, and Saul J (2001) Psychiatric morbidity and its recognition by doctors in patients with cancer. *Br. J. Cancer* **84**(8):1011–15.

Farrell MJ, Katz B, and Helme RD (1996) The impact of dementia on the pain experience. *Pain* **67**(1):7–15.

Feldman E, Mayou R, Hawton K, Ardern M, and Smith EB (1987) Psychiatric disorder in medical in-patients. *Q. J. Med.* **63**(241):405–12.

Felker B, Yazel JJ, and Short D (1996) Mortality and medical comorbidity among psychiatric patients: a review. *Psychiatr. Serv.* **47**(12):1356–63.

Foucault M (1965) *Madness and Civilisation, A History of Insanity in the Age of Reason.* Random House, New York.

Garai T and Goldsmith W (1979) Medical teamwork in a psychiatric clinic: a system that works. *Hosp. Community Psychiatry* **30**(12):848–9.

Goffman E (1968) *Stigma: Notes on the Management of Spoiled Identity.* Penguin, London.

Hanrahan P and Luchins DJ (1995) Access to hospice care for end-stage dementia patients: a national survey of hospice programs. *J. Am. Geriatr. Soc.* **43**(1):56–9.

Hayward P and Bright J (1997) Stigma and mental illness: a review and critique, *Journal of Mental Health* **6**:345–54.

Henderson M (2000) A difficult psychiatric patient. *Postgrad Med J* **76**:590–1.

Hoenig J and Hamilton J (1966) Mortality of psychiatric patients. *Acta Psychiatrica Scandinavica* **42**:349–61.

Karasu TB, Waltzman SA, Lindenmayer JP, and Buckley PJ (1980) The medical care of patients with psychiatric illness. *Hosp. Community Psychiatry* **31**(7):463–72.

Kelly BD and Shanley D (2000) Terminal illness and schizophrenia. *J. Palliat. Care* **16**(2):55–7.

Koranyi EK (1979) Morbidity and rate of undiagnosed physical illnesses in a psychiatric clinic population. *Arch. Gen. Psychiatry* **36**(4):414–19.

Lane P, Kuntupis M, MacDonald S, McCarthy P, Panke JA, Warden V, *et al.* (2003) A pain assessment tool for people with advanced Alzheimer's and other progressive dementias. *Home. Healthc. Nurse* **21**(1):32–7.

Lerner M and Miller D (1978) Just world research and the attribution process: looking back and ahead. *Psychological Bulletin* **85**:1030–51.

Maguire GP, Julier DL, Hawton KE, and Bancroft JH (1974) Psychiatric morbidity and referral on two general medical wards. *Br. Med. J.* **1**(902):268–70.

Manfredi PL, Breuer B, Meier DE, and Libow L (2003) Pain assessment in elderly patients with severe dementia. *J. Pain Symptom. Manage.* **25**(1):48–52.

Maricle R, Leung P, and Bloom JD (1987*a*) The use of DSM-III axis III in recording physical illness in psychiatric patients. *Am. J. Psychiatry* **144**(11):1484–6.

Maricle RA, Hoffman WF, Bloom JD, Faulkner LR, and Keepers GA (1987*b*) The prevalence and significance of medical illness among chronically mentally ill outpatients, *Community Ment. Health J.* **23**(2):81–90.

Marsh GW, Prochoda KP, Pritchett E, and Vojir CP (2000) Predicting hospice appropriateness for patients with dementia of the Alzheimer's type. *Appl. Nurs. Res.* **13**(4):187–96.

Massie J (1989) Depression. In Holland J and Rowland J (ed.) *Handbook of Psychooncology: Psychological Care of the Patient with Cancer.* Oxford University Press, New York.

Mayou R and Hawton K (1986) Psychiatric disorder in the general hospital. *Br. J. Psychiatry* **149**:172–90.

McConnell SD, Inderbitzin LB, and Pollard WE (1992) Primary health care in the CMHC: a role for the nurse practitioner. *Hosp. Community Psychiatry* **43**(7):724–7.

McIntyre JS and Romano J (1977) Is there a stethoscope in the house (and is it used)? *Arch. Gen. Psychiatry* **34**(10):1147–51.

Nunnally J (1961) *Popular Conceptions of Mental Health: Their Development and Change.* Rinehart and Winston, New York.

Parkes CM (1972) *Bereavement: Studies of Grief in Adult Life.* Tavistock, London.

Patel AR (1975) Attitudes towards self-poisoning *Br. Med. J.* **2**(5968):426–9.

Ramon S and Breyter C (1978) Attitudes towards self-poisoning among British and Israeli doctors and nurses in psychiatric hospitals. *Israeli Annals of Psychiatry and Related Disciplines* **16**(206):218.

Reisberg B (1988) Functional assessment staging (FAST). *Psychopharmacol. Bull.* **24**(4):653–9.

Ritchie K and Lovestone S (2002) The dementias. *Lancet* **360**:1759–66.

Saunders C (2001) The evolution of palliative care. *J. R. Soc. Med.* **94**(9):430–2.

Shuster JL, Jr. (2000) Palliative care for advanced dementia. *Clin. Geriatr. Med.* **16**(2):373–86.

Sivakumar K, Wilkinson G, Toone BK, and Greer S (1986) Attitudes to psychiatry in doctors at the end of their first post-graduate year: two-year follow-up of a cohort of medical students. *Psychol. Med.* **16**(2):457–60.

Spiess JL, Northcott CJ, Offsay JD, and Crossett JH (2002) Palliative care: something else we can do for our patients. *Psychiatr. Serv.* **53**(12):1525–6, 1529.

Talbott JA and Linn L (1978) Reactions of schizophrenics to life-threatening disease. *Psychiatr. Q.* **50**(3):218–27.

Turk DC and Okifuji A (2002) Psychological factors in chronic pain: evolution and revolution. *J. Consult Clin. Psychol.* **70**(3):678–90.

UNUM (2001) *The Cost of Sickness Absence in the UK.* UNUM, London.

Volicer BJ, Hurley A, Fabiszewski KJ, Montgomery P, and Volicer L (1993) Predicting short-term survival for patients with advanced Alzheimer's disease. *J. Am. Geriatr. Soc.* **41**(5):535–40.

Weissman DE and Matson S (1999) Pain assessment and management in the long-term care setting. *Theor. Med. Bioeth.* **20**(1):31–43.

Werneke U, Horn O, Maryon-Davis A, Hitchinson B, Wessely S, Schnaar A, *et al.* (2003) Screening for breast and cervical cancer in patients with mental illness. *Br. Med. J.* (in press).

Whately C (1959) Social attitudes toward discharged mental patients. *Social Problems* **6**:313–20.

Wilkinson DG, Toone BK, and Greer S (1983) Medical students' attitudes to psychiatry at the end of the clinical curriculum. *Psychol. Med.* **13**(3):655–8.

7

Disability

Linda McEnhill

Introduction

The rationale for discussing disability as social difference in palliative care may, at first, seem less than obvious. After all most clients accessing palliative care services are to some extent 'disabled' by their illness and palliative care practitioners have become skilful at supporting clients in the adaptation to progressive disability. Furthermore as palliative care continues to become more accessible to patients with life-limiting conditions beyond cancer (and indeed as cancer itself is transformed by improved treatments into a chronic rather than acute condition), the 'norm' will be to work with patients and their families concerning the impact of disability.

However, this chapter is based on the premise that if the attempt is made to provide palliative care without reference to the history and lived experience of the long-term (and not imminently dying) disabled population we shall do clients an injustice and be in danger of reinventing the wheel in understanding the specific issues and concerns for persons experiencing such impairments.

This aim of this chapter is to trace some of the history of disability including the development of the disabled rights movement and its response to medical and social models of disability. The focus will be on the British situation with minor reference made to the situation as it pertains in the USA.

Having laid a foundation for understanding disability per se the second part of the chapter will concentrate on palliative care of those who experience intellectual or cognitive disabilities. Recent evidence of inequity of access and treatment will be highlighted and aspects of practice outlined.

The final section of the chapter will attempt to reference areas of developing literature and practice in response to the previously identified challenges and give guidance on developing responsive services.

A social history of disability

In ancient history disability was regarded with suspicion, later through the eyes of Judaeo/Christian traditions as a consequence of personal sin. In the 20th century medicine and the medical model has provided the main arena in which disability has been defined and 'treated'.

Medicine traditionally describes disability as a specific impairment or impairments of physical, sensory, or mental abilities. In Britain this affects 10% of the population. Whilst many disabled people are not 'ill' they have experienced the impact of a medical model, characterized by Bilton as one where disease is seen as a temporary organic state to be cured or eradicated by reactive medical intervention without reference to non-organic factors (Bilton in Marks 2001). Thus many disabled people are consigned to a perceptual ability/disability binary in the thinking of others and a consequent assumption that disabled people are merely dependent recipients of care received from omnipotent non-disabled deliverers (Barnes in Marks 2001). Critics of the medical model see it as a form of social control which de-skills, labels, and creates passivity whilst refusing to acknowledge its own value base. Such a model impacts not only on the environment and behaviour of the disabled but also on construction of their personal identity. The continual 'objectifying gaze' of medical interventions asserts that the disabled person is not acceptable as they are but must be 'fixed' or 'put right' (Illich in Marks 2001). Sinason describes how this often results in practices which distance the healthcare professional from understanding the disabled person's emotional world and renders them incapable of acknowledging their painful experiences (Sinason 1992).

It was not until the 1970s-80s that the disability rights movement began, typically, Marks says, lagging behind movements of other minority groups. The movement began first in America with an emphasis on services and consumer rights promoted by a large group of young ex- servicemen disabled in the Vietnam War. In Britain the movement was influenced more strongly by socialism and so had a stronger emphasis on the organization of work and property.

In learning disability an equivalent movement took place, influenced by the concept of 'normalization' which was being simultaneously developed (Wolfensberger 1972). Normalization asserted that the learning disabled had rights to equivalent life opportunities of non-disabled people. This movement also had an American origin in the influential concept of 'self-advocacy' introduced by the 'People First' group when they visited England (Sinason 1992).

At the heart of these movements was a concern not only for equity of civil rights but to gain full 'cultural citizenship', rather than be recipients of special privileges. From this the 'social model' of disability was developed which defines disability not as a *tragic aberration afflicting a minority of people*' (Marks 2001) but as the effect of an environment which discriminates against and disables certain 'impaired individuals'. Therefore state institutions such as education, social services, and the economy have a determinative role in shaping the oppression of disabled people.

Certain social theorists concentrated on the role which industrialization played in creating disabling environments (by demanding a uniformly able-bodied workforce it disenfranchised and segregated the disabled) (Finkelstein in Marks 2001). Others concentrated on the impact of visible symbols such as architecture, which not only bars access to the disabled but at a subconscious level suggests they do not exist:

'*Design aesthetics reflect certain idealised assumptions about the inhabitants and users of the built environment*' (Marks 2001) or which, when adapting buildings for access in conflict with the original design aesthetic, suggests disability '*is something which cannot be harmoniously included in the able bodied world*' (Marks 2001).

Whilst most disabled people would see the social model as an improvement on the medical model, it is not without its critics. Some have argued that it is reductionist in not accounting for the complexity of inter-relationships in a disabled person's life. A person is not only embodied as a person with a disability but also as a person with colour, culture, gender, race, and sexual preference. The social model by concentrating solely on disability leaves no room for these aspects of personhood. Others have criticized the model for its allegiance to capitalist values and its consequent primacy of attention on work and independence and thereby prioritizing of disabilities of mobility over the spectrum of limitations which disabled people experience.

One of the most damning criticisms of the model is the charge of discrimination against people with intellectual impairments. Apsis suggests that people with learning difficulties face discrimination in the disability movement stemming in part from the latter group's fear of being labelled 'stupid, thick, mental, and mad, by the non-disabled public' (Apsis in Marks 2001).

Archaeology of disability

Alongside the social history of disability a parallel history exists. This history is one of thoughts and feelings that undergird the responses which the disabled person encounters in society at both a micro and macro level. Foucault describes the analysis of this underbelly as an 'archaeology', exploring human beings 'problematizations of themselves, their world and their actions'. Its importance lies in revealing the fundamental issues and problems in terms of which individuals confront their existence (Gutton 2001). This is predominantly the experience of 'difference', of being treated as 'other'. As we endeavour to understand the world of disability it is important to reflect on the experience of difference in this context and its implications for our practice.

From the earliest times Greek and Roman societies practised infanticide on sickly or deformed children. In the middle ages superstitious beliefs led to the persecution of disabled people and in Western religious communities there has been a long association between disability as the consequence of personal sin, evil, or the practice of witchcraft (Marks 2001). However, as a more medically enlightened culture developed a new concept also evolved, that of eugenics. This is the idea that to preserve the purity of the human genetic pool one must prevent reproduction by genetically inferior members; a concept influenced by Darwinian thinking but held alongside a belief that it was the duty of those that have the power to intervene in the natural processes so to do, resulting in medical sterilization of those who were considered to be feeble minded or criminally insane (Wolfensberger 1987). By 1920 there were laws in 25 American states legislating for the compulsory sterilization of people in these categories and by 1958 60,000 Americans had been forcibly sterilized (Hubbard in Marks 2001).

The most prevalent understanding of eugenic philosophy is in its use against Jewish people in Nazi Germany. Less publicity has been given to the number of disabled people who were killed in the holocaust or to the fact that exterminations of the disabled continued to be carried out for up to 6 months after the liberation of the concentration camps. These deaths required the active or passive co-operation of doctors in completing the documentation required informing the authorities of the existence of a disabled person to be 'euthanized' or in carrying out the euthanasia itself. Yet Gallagher demonstrates that no doctors were prosecuted for war crimes against disabled people (Gallagher in Marks 2001).

Alongside eugenic thinking the influence of utilitarianism has impacted on attitudes towards disabled people. This is the idea that those who are dependent on others, or who experience high levels of suffering have lives that are not worth living. Proponents of this 'myth' of independence (e.g. Glover 1988) see physical and mental autonomy to be the defining qualities of personhood and the basis on which people's lives should be sustained (Glover 1988). Such attitudes are expressed concretely in the practices of amniocentesis, abortion, and euthanasia.

Wolfensberger suggests that in each of these practices is expressed society's '*death wish*' towards people with disabilities (Wolfensberger in Sinason 1992). Sinason explores the psychological impact of this message that one is better not to have been born or better to have died. She shows that even significantly intellectually impaired individuals understand the meaning of the word amniocentesis and that society's hostility towards disability may result in people with learning disabilities developing harmful defences (secondary handicaps) expressed in behaviours such as the '*handicapped smile*' (Sinason 1992).

Many parents-to-be would not be able to contemplate the birth of a child with a disability and where such is diagnosed then termination may be carried out up until the 40th week of pregnancy (in other situations the cut off is 20 weeks). However, parents who do give birth to a disabled child recount vividly the pervasiveness of this death wish, within a society which cannot celebrate the birth (Boston 1981, 1994) and even within themselves (Hannam 1975). There are also, however, many accounts of the depth of affectional bonds that may be established between parent and child based on unconditional love rather than any utilitarian values. Whilst one cannot underestimate the complexity of the issues involved in the decision to abort a child, or pronounce judgement on the moral status of such a decision, it is important to remember Wolfensberger's caution that a judgement about 'quality of life' may become a presupposition about the 'value of life'.

Robert's story

Robert was twenty-one when he was diagnosed as having a testicular teratoma and referred to the cancer centre. As a result of his learning disability it was assumed that he could not consent to treatment and therefore would not undergo potentially curative surgery and chemotherapy.

Robert's key-worker and the medical social worker helped him to understand his treatment options and express his wishes, which were documented in his case notes. As a result it was decided that Robert should have chemotherapy after his surgery. The treatment team leader's response was: 'What a shame to put him through this'.

Rachel's story

Rachel's carers had taken her to her GP many times over a period of months when she consistently complained of stomach pains. One weekend she was admitted to the local hospital having gone into bowel obstruction. Surgery revealed that Rachel had previously ruptured her bowel and that it had subsequently healed over; she was also found to have two small secondary tumours on her liver. It was decided (contrary to 'normal' practice) that these would not be treated with surgery or chemotherapy. Rachel, aged forty-two, died nine months later.

Morris makes a similar case in exploring court responses to requests for voluntary euthanasia (assisted suicide) from disabled people. She suggests that disabled people are considered to be making a rational request purely on the basis of the fact that they have a disability, without recourse to other disabled people in arriving at such a decision. She cites a number of cases where the social circumstances lead her to ask ' … is the wish to die a so-called rational response to physical disability? Or is it a desperate response to isolated oppression?' Chillingly she suggests that '*No mental disturbance or emotional trauma is deemed necessary to explain the rejection of life by a disabled person. Instead their physical disability is taken as sufficient grounds to want to die*' (Morris in Davey *et al.* 2000).

Todd picks up this theme and shows that often the birth of a person with a disability (here specifically learning disability) is treated as bereavement and that the model of counselling usually offered to parents reflects this. Todd links this to the paucity of literature on or concern with the dying experience of people with learning disabilities. He sees the personal tragedy model of disability influencing the response to such a death resulting in it often being perceived of as a 'release'. The implications of this for the parents' bereavement and how the deceased will be remembered have yet to be fully explored (Todd 2002).

Legislation and equity of access

Since 1981, the International Year of Disabled Persons, the tenor of thinking, expressed in UK legislation, has taken on an increasingly holistic tone. Rather than disability being described purely in medical terms there is an incorporation of the social. Participation as a full citizen in society is expressed as a fundamental aim. Despite legislation there are still many instances of discrimination on the basis of disability, most frequently these are demonstrated with regard to employment. The evidence of discrimination with regard to inequity of healthcare has also been well demonstrated, this is especially so in the case of people with learning disabilities.

Healthcare policy and people with learning disabilities

The Department of Health's '*The Health of the Nation: a strategy for people with learning difficulties*' (1995) identified 3 elements of good healthcare for people with learning disabilities, these were:

◆ Health Prevention

◆ Early detection of illness

◆ Good care in ill health.

This was followed in 1998 by '*Signposts for Success*' the Department of Health guidance on commissioning and providing such services. However the Mencap report '*The NHS—Health for all?'(1998)* demonstrated that in terms of these three elements the NHS poorly served people with learning disabilities. This was most obvious in terms of cancer screening services.

Table 7.1 Mencap 1998

	% Eligible 'Ordinary' Public Screened	% Eligible Learning Disabled Screened
Breast cancer screening	76%	50% (of which 52% formal care, 17% living at home)
Cervical cancer screening	85%	17% in formal care, 3% living at home

Following this report, work undertaken by the Department of Health in developing guidelines for '*Good Practice in Breast and Cervical Screening for Women with Learning Disabilities*' (2000), produced not only information for professionals, but also pictorial information for women with learning disabilities.

It remains to be seen how much improvement has been made in the healthcare of people with learning disabilities. Certainly the findings presented in the Mencap report '*No ordinary life*' (2001) suggest that the burden of care still rests heavily on informal carers. This research found that carers of people with profound and multiple disabilities spent on average 18 hours per day caring for their son or daughter, were woken on average 3 times per night, but only received, on average, 20 minutes per day assistance from support services (Mencap 2001).

The '*Valuing People*' white paper (2001*b*) explores (Chapter six) the healthcare needs of people with learning disabilities and makes a number of recommendations. Some of the aims are surprisingly low—for example that all people with a learning disability be registered with a GP by 2004. However other aims such as access to healthcare facilitators, health action plans and annual health checks aim to reduce inequalities. This echoes the findings of the Scottish Executive report '*The same as you?*'(2000) and is reinforced in a Scottish national review of nurses and midwives caring for people with learning disabilities '*Promoting Health, Supporting Inclusion*' (2003). Potentially these policies offer a positive way forward in equalizing healthcare generally and palliative care specifically for this client group but only if effective working partnerships across the boundaries of learning disability, health and palliative care services can be forged.

Palliative care access and people with learning disabilities

Before we leave this section we pause briefly to consider the little research that has been carried out specifically with regard to cancer and palliative care services.

Whilst acknowledging that problems of access do not appear to lie so much with palliative care providers as with referrers to their services, two pieces of research deserve note:

The first of these (Hogg *et al.* 2001) researched the subject of cancer care and people with learning disabilities. Hogg explored published studies of the incidence of cancer in people with learning disabilities and also interviewed current learning-disabled cancer patients about their experience of cancer services. The findings are probably provisional due to sample sizes and the inherent difficulties of working from previously published material. However in terms of palliative care, the findings though largely positive, were that people with learning disabilities accessing palliative care were unlikely to be offered the full range of services. This was especially so in the case of complementary therapies and hospice day care placements, which were rarely offered.

The second study carried out by the Salomon's Centre, University of Kent at Canterbury (Brown *et al.* 2003), reflected Hogg's findings concerning the importance of good community working relationships and role clarity in determining positive patient outcomes. However, in mapping the care received by persons suffering from dementia and persons suffering from a malignancy there are unsurprising results. Those suffering from dementia had less support from secondary health care (and virtually none from palliative care) whilst those suffering from a terminal malignancy were well supported by the secondary health care services reducing the burden on informal carers and residential settings. This is an important consideration for palliative care services that wish to increase accessibility to the learning disabled population as, given the predisposition of people with Downs syndrome to early onset dementia, it is in this area that learning disability services may wish for support.

Issues for practice

Some of these are more relevant to the care of people with intellectual disabilities. However, the template at the end of the chapter is intended to be of relevance in developing services for all people with a disability. The emphasis is placed on emotional and spiritual aspects of care.

Communication

In palliative care communication is key and in the advent of communication training for doctors palliative care has been an important development. However, in the care of people with disabilities, its importance is paramount and the core team may have to enlarge to incorporate the skills of speech therapy or to make extended use of occupational therapy in working with assistive communication aids and techniques. Our colleagues who have worked in the areas of stroke, motor neurone disease, and multiple sclerosis may be best placed to enable us to find creative ways to communicate when physical speech is not possible. In learning disability, communication presents potentially more complex challenges. Some clients may not use verbal communication and although they understand spoken language, may convey that understanding in sign language such as Makaton, or they may use an idiosyncratic sign language understood only by them and closest family members or carers. Most complex is the situation where the learning disabled adult uses spoken language but their conceptual world is unevenly developed and many of their concepts are as one would expect of quite a young child. This is especially so in terms of whether the client is capable of abstract thought or whether they are at a developmental stage, intellectually, where they are predominately a concrete or literal thinker. The often proficient use of spoken language may then belie very underdeveloped concepts in terms of time, personal identity, of illness, its progression and of death itself. Consequently some of our models for breaking bad news (Maguire and Faulkner 1988; Buckman 1992) will require significant adaptation to communicate with someone who does not understand the subtlety of the 'warning shot', or the need to ask questions to get the information required.

Equally the need to gain consent for treatment from someone with mismatched understanding and performance skills is a task which tries the abilities of the most skilled practitioner. It is important to remember that:

- Everyone should be presumed to be competent unless proven otherwise (i.e. not presumed to be incompetent)

- That people are not universally competent (i.e. it is possible to be competent to consent to the removal of a painful decayed tooth whilst perhaps not being competent to consent to palliative chemotherapy)

- That no one can consent to treatment on behalf of another adult (incapacitated or not)

- That incapacity in and of itself is not grounds for refusing to give medical treatment (doctors are required to act in the 'best interests' of a patient irrespective of their ability to consent—though the process is slightly more complicated than the statement!).

The Adults with Incapacity (Scotland) Act 2000 has clarified this situation and the Department of Health guidelines are also helpful (DoH 2001a). Given the conceptual difficulties outlined above important information and informed consent may take many sessions to both convey and confirm.

Diagnosis and treatment

Inequity of access to screening services has already been highlighted and the implications for diagnosis are obvious. However, this is not the only difficulty. It has been shown consistently that many people with learning disabilities fail to be diagnosed (especially with a malignancy) until their disease has progressed beyond hope of curative treatment.

The reasons for this are complex, involving the care setting in which people live (i.e. whether or not staff or family members have the skills or training to recognize the significance of early symptoms) and the way in which illness is communicated (more likely behaviourally than verbally). Of equal concern is the phenomenon of 'diagnostic overshadowing' where there is an over attribution of the learning disability in assessment of illness. This leads the physician to conclude that whatever is presented or reported to her is just 'part of the learning disability' (Howells in O'Hara and Sperlinger 1997). This situation is exacerbated in the high proportion of gastric malignancies reported in this group (26% of total malignancies), which are notoriously difficult to diagnose in any case (Hogg 2001).

A lack of awareness and training in learning disability amongst health professionals leaves this group vulnerable not only to failure to diagnose serious illness but, the literature suggests, in subsequent treatment and control of symptoms (Lindop and Read 2000; Astor 2001; Tuffrey-Wijne 2003). The groundbreaking NHS Beacon work by Regnard and the learning disability team at Northgate and Prudhoe hospital in the UK in developing palliative care services for people with learning disabilities has therefore been especially useful (Northgate Palliative Care Team 2001; Regnard *et al.* 2002, 2003). Confronted with numerous anecdotal accounts of people not receiving adequate symptom control, and of the powerlessness of their carers to convince healthcare professionals of their clients' needs, they have developed the concept of LOC, the Language of Observable Communication.

This concept asserts that people with learning disabilities, even without speech, do communicate, and that we are deficient in trying to understand the true meaning of that communication. It is suggested that this communication (which is mainly behavioural) constitutes a language in its own right. To interpret it we require understanding of the baseline communication (i.e. how someone presents when they are happy and pain free) so that we can evaluate the significance of any changes which are expressed. The team has also developed a communication tool in assessing distress (the DisDAT tool) which would be useful not only for learning disabled clients but for any client where verbal communication is difficult.

At the end of life

There is an extensive literature on the care of the dying from both medical and psychosocial standpoints. It is presumed that this is equally applicable to people with physical and intellectual disabilities. Concerning the person with learning disabilities there are additional issues related to the ability to conceptualize death and whether they operate in contexts where awareness of death is a possibility.

In terms of understanding death it has been established that a complete understanding involves many aspects but the essential components are understanding that death is universal, inevitable, permanent, as well as something about causes of death. These concepts are gained within a developmental framework and therefore for a person with a learning disability will be related to their level of cognitive ability. However, research has also shown that the concept of death may be less complete depending on whether someone has lived in a long-term institution (Lipe-Godson and Goebel 1983). In terms of the present learning-disabled palliative care population this is an important consideration.

It has been demonstrated that people with intellectual disabilities exist mostly in 'closed awareness contexts' where information is not shared openly between staff and service users (Glaser and Strauss 1964). The tendency to infantalize and concern regarding the client's concept of time, make it likely that a person with a learning disability may not have been informed of their impending death. In this situation the palliative care professional's task of facilitating shared awareness may be complex and met with understandable resistance from learning disability colleagues. However, Todd (citing Wilson) reminds us that such knowledge is vital for the client in enabling them to have some control over the manner of their demise (Wilson in Todd 2002).

Confronted with an awareness of the terminal nature of their condition many patients express concern that they should neither die alone, in pain or in indignity. This mirrors my own experience of working with terminally ill learning disabled people but in addition the concern is consistently expressed in the need to know that they will be remembered.

Todd writing about the lack of evidence relating to the remembrance of deceased people with learning disabilities relates this to the 'social death', which they may have experienced throughout their lives (Todd 2002). This is most aptly summed up in his words elsewhere when he asks '*What type of ancestors do people with learning disabilities make?*' Whether due to an awareness of society's negation or not, questions are asked of helpers such as '*You'll miss me when I'm gone?*' (Expressed simultaneously as a statement and a question). Or in the request for lots of flowers at the funeral because people who are loved and remembered have lots of flowers. For one woman it was expressed as sadness at her lack of children and significant relationships in her life when she said:

> When I'm gone there will be nothing to remind anyone of me. When my mother dies they'll know she existed because of me, but when I am gone it will be like I was a [photographic] negative, like I never existed at all.

Perhaps here palliative care has a significant contribution to make. Using techniques such as formal life review and combining it with concrete tools like life story books may enable patients to undertake essential preparatory work and be reassured by some symbol of remembering. It is important for remaining service users that in facilitation of adjustment to 'the changed environment' all signs of the deceased's existence are not removed so that in remembering they will know that they too will be remembered.

In this context the spiritual care of people with learning disabilities is important. The work of Young and Swinton has done much to improve our understanding (Young 1990; Swinton 1999, 2001). Swinton enlightens us to the significance of 'friendship' as the vehicle by which spirituality is commonly conceived. I suspect that combining this metaphor with the concerns expressed above, the resulting idea of a deity as one who is a 'friend' who always (eternally) remembers may have something to offer people struggling to contemplate the end of their physical lives.

Bereavement

Sinason's innovative work, in the late 1970s, revolutionized therapeutic thinking concerning people with learning disabilities.

> 'Firstly, we concluded that no handicap in itself meant that a patient could not make use of therapy. There could be emotional intelligence left intact and rich regardless of how crippled performance intelligence was' (Sinason 1992).

This belief undergirds the seminal bereavement work undertaken by practitioners Hollins and Sireling (1989*a*, *b*), Oswin (1991), and Cathcart (1994, 1996), and recently developed by Read (2000) and Blackman (2000, 2003). Bereavement work with this group, though essentially simple, and at heart creative, is not without complexity. The complexity arises both in the social situations in which the bereavement occurs and because of the conceptual and communication issues already discussed.

The profusion of social and psychological losses experienced by the person with learning disabilities generally exceeds those that are experienced by the 'ordinary' person. The significance of this for traditional bereavement risk analysis is not conclusive, but is suggestive of the need to err on the side of offering more rather than less support. The service situations in which many people with learning disabilities live are also not conducive to good bereavement care. As a result of staff not being trained to recognize or understand bereavement, there is evidence of it being missed, misinterpreted or made worse by the cumulative losses which service responses often initiate. For example Oswin found that a person with learning disabilities living in the community when their carer died was on average likely to be moved 5 times within the first year of the bereavement. The literature also highlights how often bereaved people with learning disabilities are denied access to the rites of passage which are generally accepted as facilitative of healthy grief (Oswin 1991; Hollins and Esterhuyzen 1997).

Equally generic bereavement supporters may not have an adequate understanding of learning disability and consequently be uncomfortable using a developmental model of grief counselling or behavioural techniques like guided mourning (McEnhill 2000). They may not be prepared for the behavioural expression of the grief (for example physical searching behaviour) or find it difficult to work with someone who does not use speech. Work by Read and Blackman is helpful in suggesting new ways of working and adapting standard models (Read 2000; Blackman 2000, 2003). Evaluating interventions requires concrete input from service users and those close to them to look at the impact which 'therapy' had. The importance of offering such help (however unskilled) cannot be over emphasized as figures for depression and challenging behaviour (including self-injury) post bereavement are alarmingly high. However, bereaved people with learning disabilities are still more likely to be offered behaviour modification programmes than bereavement counselling (McEvoy 1989).

There is an urgent need for bereavement theory as it relates to people with learning disabilities to take seriously the impact of newer models of grief including Stroebe (1993), Wortman *et al.* (1993) and Walter (1996). The poverty of information which many learning disabled people have about their own lives, combined with a diminished ability to retain a mental record of their history, mean that we need to find alternative ways to enable people to tell 'their' story and to find an appropriate place for the deceased within it.

Anna's story

Anna had been visiting her parental home when her father became unwell. Her stepmother discovered that he had collapsed behind the bathroom door. Anna was sent to the garden and the door into the house locked. During the three hours that Anna was in the garden the ambulance and police services were called and her father's body removed from the house. Although Anna attended the funeral the coffin was closed and she never saw her father again. Six months later when referred for bereavement counselling Anna's self injurious behaviour had escalated to her placing her hands onto the ignited electric rings of a cooker.

Andrew's story

Andrew was referred by a psychiatrist for bereavement counselling when discharged from hospital after a severe depression in which Andrew gave up eating and drinking. Andrew had witnessed the fatal injury of two of his flatmates who he had known for twenty years. Although keen to undergo counselling the care staff blocked the referral believing the 'bereavement' to be Andrew's excuse for his bad behaviour as he only ever mentioned it when destroying the kitchen.

Education and staff support

The final section of this chapter explores education and staff support. Of all the areas of difference between learning disability and palliative care services, these are the most distinct. In the United Kingdom the palliative care work force is amongst the most qualified and educated of any, whilst the British learning disability workforce is younger, less experienced and 75% of it are unqualified (DoH 2001b). Despite this, many learning disability workers confront daily significant loss, emotional pain, and physical challenge. In contrast to the palliative care force they receive little in the way of clinical supervision and due to budget restraints are not eligible for the vast range of educational opportunities which palliative care professionals access.

However in response to the crisis in social care the government has set a target for training (similar to the NVQ system) learning disability staff (DoH 2001b). The LDAF (Learning Disability Awards Framework) provides a baseline in holistic client care. This presents an opportunity for both learning disability and for palliative care in being able to provide and access education in the palliative care approach.

Ordinarily palliative care communities are not given to thinking of themselves as having an abundance of resources. However in building partnerships with community learning disability providers they certainly are the richer partner and have much to offer. Our experience at St. Nicholas Hospice (in Bury St. Edmunds, England) is that in return for offering expertise, we have been greeted with a hunger for learning and a willingness to put into practice and on some occasions mini-buses full of staff from care homes to attend an afternoon session. The very real value of this work has been in the partnerships that have been generated and an increased ability for community practitioners to care for their client in their own home. Opposite is a table of this education provision provided within the hospice presently.

Conclusion

The final word in conclusion of this chapter concerns partnership. Whilst there is already a strong knowledge and skill base within palliative care to provide sensitive services for people with disabilities, there are also obvious deficits most particularly in the care of people with learning disabilities. The percentage of the population with learning disabilities is around 2% although the figure is predicted to grow by 1% of its total annually for the foreseeable future. The number of presenting palliative care cases, at any given time, is therefore likely to be small. For many this will be the justification for taking no action, despite the wisdom that '*Those who refuse to learn from history are condemned to repeat it*'. However, neither is there justification for the creation of yet more specialist posts for example a lung cancer specialist nurse for people with learning disabilities, fragmenting knowledge and care and conflicting with the spirit of the ('Valuing People') white paper (DoH 2001*b*).

It is clear that if services are to be responsive to the complex needs of this client group they have to be able to react quickly to referrals and therefore require access to identified and established resources. One of the most profitable ways ahead is likely to be the creation of link-workers as a team resource and co-ordination between the different care partners. The work being undertaken by the cancer charity, Macmillan Cancer Relief, in employing learning disability nurses to some palliative care nursing posts, may be foundational in this development (Murphy 2003).

There are also a number of innovative projects throughout the United Kingdom. However, as most of these are Lottery funded and uncoordinated their long-term contributions are uncertain. Never before has there been such a need to network and build partnerships if we are to be responsive to client need. This is the role which any hospice can begin to undertake whether it seeks to do this through a national organization such as The National Network for the Palliative Care of People with Learning Disabilities or whether it seeks to do so at a very local level using the resources of its education department. The important thing is that we must do it or face the danger, as Todd says, of discriminating against this group not only in their living but also in their dying and beyond (Todd 2002).

Table 7.2 Palliative care and learning disability education (St. Nicholas Hospice 2003)

Title	Duration	Learners	Cost
Practice updates	Weekly afternoon session	Hospice staff and volunteers, hospital and community staff	Without charge
Intro. to palliative care and people with learning disabilities	1 afternoon 6 monthly	Hospice staff and volunteers, hospital, community staff, nursing and care home staff	Without charge
Loss and bereavement and people with learning disabilities	3 days	District nurses, hospice staff, nursing care homes, clergy	With charge
Palliative care and people with learning disabilities	3 days	District nurses, Hospice staff, Nursing and care homes, Community staff	With charge
LDAF (Learning Disability Awards Framework) writing and delivering module on Palliative Care	Several ½ Day sessions	Learning Disability Service	With charge
Conference/Study day	1 Day annually	Joint award students, community practitioners	Some free places for students and unwaged
Consultancy/Supervision/ Staff Support	As required	Carers of people with learning disability	Free if part of package of care.
Joint social work and learning disability award placement	90 Day Placement	Joint Award Students	With charge

Table 7.3 Framework for achieving accessible and appropriate palliative care services for people with disabilities (adapted from 'Good Practices in Palliative Care by Oliviere, Hargreaves and Monroe 1998)

	Principle	Practice
Mission statement	Commitment to equality in value base and stated aims	Staff and service users aware. Mission statement displayed with pictorial symbols.
Policy and procedures	Management committed. Equal opportunities policy	Joint understanding of policy and procedures. Independent advocates used.
Staff selection	Staff matching ethos. Community participation as volunteers.	Service users involved in selection of staff and volunteers. Positive selection of staff and volunteers with disabilities. Selection of staff from diverse background and training (e.g. Mental Handicap Nursing).
Training	Skilled workforce	People with disabilities involved in staff training. Link-worker posts developed.
Environment	User friendly, hospitable trust	Furnishings friendly but practicable. Use of colour as cues for people with problems of memory and orientation.
Written material	Good communication	Communications in written, pictorial and audio versions. Ability to involve Makaton or British Sign Language (BSL) signer when appropriate
Language	Good communication	Train staff in LOC (Language of Observable Communication). Recruit signers from minority ethnic groups. Involve advocates and health facilitators.
Community development	Trust building, equal access	Link with local disability services.
Disability monitoring	Information on those currently accessing	Record on database and investigate referral patterns. Monitor staff training needs

Patient Notes	Accurate information to plan care	Initial baseline behavioural/communication assessment to be undertaken jointly with disability care staff/family. Including language used, preferred name. Dietary, religious requirements. Normal daily pattern
Resources	Patient comfort	Availability of range of entertainment resources appropriate to the disability (e.g. large screen TV rather than small bedside). Consider sensory stimulation materials
Diet, Physical Care	Good care	Ensure disabled clients are offered full range of services including day care and complementary therapies. Awareness of feeding difficulties
Pastoral Care	Respect for individuals	Develop or access local team of clergy familiar with and responsive to the spiritual needs of people with disabilities.
Personal Care	Individuality and respect	Understanding of patients' background including issues relating to institutional care or abuse. Respect choice
Family and Community	Support for patient's network	Understand culture of family/service setting and the need to support possibly a wide range of 'family' members
Bereavement	Prevention	Stimulate awareness of specific bereavement needs and techniques. Work with community counsellors to meet the same.
Education	Resource good care	Offer education on a number of levels including update sessions, consultancy and student placements. Develop up to date resource library for sharing with community colleagues. Encourage involvement at national as well as local level.
Feedback and Evaluation	Service improvement	Consult both individuals and groups using a range of evaluative techniques. Involve people with disabilities in service development and service user forums

References

Astor R (2001) Detecting pain in people with profound learning disabilities. *Nursing Times* **97**:38–39.

Blackman N (2003) *Loss and Learning Disability.* London Worth Publishing Ltd.

Blackman N (ed.) (2000) *Living with Loss: Helping People with Learning Disabilities Cope with Bereavement and Loss.* Pavilion Publishing, Brighton.

Boston S (1981) *Will, My Son: The Life and Death of a Mongol Child.* Pluto Press Ltd, London.

Boston S (1994) *Too Deep for Tears.* Pandora Harper Collins, London.

Brown H, Burns S, and Flynn M (2003) *Dying Matters.* London Salomons Centre Kent & Foundation for People with Learning Disabilities, London.

Buckman R (1992) *How to Break Bad news: A Guide for Healthcare Professionals.* Papermac, London.

Cathcart F (1994). *Understanding Death & Dying* (Books 1–3) Kidderminster. BILD.

Cathcart F (1996) Death and People with Learning Disabilities: Interventions to Support Clients and Carers. Parts 1 and 2 *Bereavement Care* **15**:7–9, 20–22.

Davey B, Gray A, and Seale C (2000) *Health and Disease: A Reader.* Open University Press, Buckingham.

Department of Health (1995) *The Health of The Nation: A Strategy for People with Learning Disability'* 1995. HMSO, London.

Department of Health (1998) *Signposts for Success in Commissioning and Providing Health Services for People with Learning Disabilities.* Wetherby. Department of Health.

Department of Health (2000) *Good Practice in Breast and Cervical Screening of Women with Learning Disabilities.* London Department of Health.

Department of Health (2001*a*). *Seeking Consent: Working with People with Learning Disabilities.* London. Department of Health.

Department of Health (2001*b*) *'Valuing People: a New Strategy for Learning Disability for the 21st Century'.* White Paper. London. Department of Health.

Glaser BG and Strauss AL (1964) Awareness contexts and social interaction. *American Sociological Review* **29**:669–79.

Glover J (1988) *Causing Deaths and Saving Lives.* Penguin Books, Middlesex.

Gutton G (2001) *French Philosophy in the Twentieth Century.* Cambridge University Press, Cambridge.

Hannam C (1975) *Parents and Mentally Handicapped Children.* Bristol Classical Press, Bristol.

Hogg J, Northfield J, and Turnbull J (2001) *Cancer and People with Learning Disabilities: The Evidence from Published Studies and Experiences from Cancer Services.* BILD, Kidderminster.

Hollins S and Sireling L (1989*a*) *When Mum Died.* St. George's Medical School, London.

Hollins S and Sireling L (1989*b*) *When Dad Died.* St. George's Medical School, London.

Hollins S and Esterhuyzen A (1997) Bereavement and grief in adults with learning disabilities. *British Journal of Psychiatry* **170**:497–501.

Lindop P and Read S (2000) District nurses needs: palliative care for people with learning disabilities. *International Journal of Palliative Nursing* **6**:117–22.

Lipe-Godson P and Goebel B (1983) Perception of age and death in mentally retarded adults. *Mental Retardation* **21**:68–75.

McEnhill L (2000) Guided mourning interventions (Chpt1). In Blackman N (ed.) *Living with Loss: Helping People with Learning Disabilities Cope with Bereavement and Loss.* Pavilion Publishing, Brighton.

McEvoy J (1989) Investigating the concept of death in adults who are mentally handicapped. *British Journal of Mental Subnormality* **35**(2):69.

Maguire P and Faulkner A (1988) How to do it: communicate with cancer patients and their relatives. *British Medical Journal* **297**:907–24.

Marks D (2001) *Disability: Controversial Debates and Psychosocial Perspectives.* Routledge, London.

MENCAP (1998) *The NHS: Health for all? People with Learning Disabilities and Healthcare.* Mencap National Centre, London.

MENCAP (2001) *No Ordinary Life: the Support Needs of Families Caring for Children and Adults with Profound and Multiple Learning Disabilities.* Mencap National Headquarters, London.

Murphy A (2003) Supporting Special Needs. *Macmillan Voice* **27**:8.

Northgate Palliative Care Team DisDAT (2001) Northgate and Prudhoe Trust.

O'Hara A and Sperlinger A (1997)(ed.) *Adults with Learning Disabilities: A Practical Approach for Health Professionals.* John Wiley and Sons, Chichester.

Oliviere D, Hargreaves R, and Monroe B (1998) *Good Practices in Palliative Care.* Ashgate Publishing Ltd, Aldershot.

Oswin M (1991) *Am I Allowed to Cry?* Souvenir Press Ltd, London.

Read S (2000) Creative ways of working when exploring the bereavement counselling process (Chpt 2). In Blackman N (ed.) *Living with Loss: Helping People with Learning Disabilities Cope with Bereavement and Loss.* Pavilion Publishing, Brighton.

Regnard C, Gibson L, and Jenson C (2002) *Clip Worksheets.* Radcliffe Medical Press, Oxford.

Regnard C, Matthews D, Gibson L, and Clarke C (2003) Difficulties in identifying distress and its causes in people with severe communication problems. *International Journal of Palliative Nursing* **9**(4):173–6.

Scottish Executive (2000) The same as you: review of services for people with learning disabilities. Scotland.

Scottish Executive (2003) Promoting Health–Supporting Inclusion. Scotland.

Sheldon F (1997) *Psychosocial Palliative Care: Good Practice in the Care of the Dying and Bereaved.* Thornes (Publishers) Ltd, Cheltenham.

Sinason V (1992) *Mental Handicap and the Human Condition: New Approaches from the Tavistock.* Free Association Books Ltd., London.

Stroebe M.S and Stroebe W (1993) *Handbook of Bereavement: Theory, Research and Intervention.* Cambridge University Press, Cambridge.

Swinton J (1999) *Building a Church for Strangers: Theology, Church and Learning Disabilities.* Edinburgh. Contact Pastoral Trust.

Swinton J (2001) *A Space to Listen: Meeting the Spiritual Needs of People with Learning Disabilities.* The Mental Health Foundation, London.

Todd S (2002) Death does not become us: the absence of death and dying in intellectual disability research. *Journal of Gerontological Social Work* **38**: 225–39.

Tuffrey-Wijne I (2003) The palliative care needs of people with intellectual disabilities: a literature review. *Palliative Medicine* 17(8):55–62.

Walter T (1996) A new model of grief. *Mortality* 1:7–25.

Wolfensberger W (1972) *Normalisation.* Toronto National Institute of Mental Retardation.

Wolfensberger W (1987) *The New Genocide of Handicapped and Afflicted People.* Syracuse University Division of Special Education and Rehabilitation, Syracuse.

Wortman C, Silver R, and Kessler R (1993) Adjustment to bereavement. In Stroebe MS and Stroebe W (ed.) *Handbook of Bereavement: Theory, Practice and Intervention.* University of Cambridge Press, Cambridge.

Young F (1990) *Face to Face: A Narrative Study in the Theology of Suffering.* T&T Clark, Edinburgh.

8

Abuse

Maggie Draper and Chris Wood

If you were to eavesdrop on any gathering of palliative care staff, and especially those who work in the community, you would hear story after story of concerns, uneasiness, and anxieties about people who live in squalor or fear.

These stories would include: the person who is trapped upstairs in a tiny bedroom (because to have a bed or commode downstairs would be untidy, and unacceptable), to the cases of severe self neglect; misuse and manipulation of medication or fluids by carers; financial exploitation by the homeless family member who suddenly volunteers to be a carer; the ill, cognitively impaired, and disinhibited patient who makes uncharacteristic aggressive sexual demands of their spouse; the paid carer who is untrained and disinterested; the family reconciliation when wills are made or altered.

What is striking about the retelling of these tales is the anxieties of the workers, their sense of disgust and feelings of helplessness, their frustration about not being able to provide a solution, their indignation about this happening to the dying, and the challenge to their aspirations to help people have a dignified death. Rights and values of patients and their carers may conflict, a patient's mental capacity may be difficult to assess, family secrets may be powerful, and always, when working with the dying, time is short.

The abuse of vulnerable adults, as well as being physical or sexual, can also be emotional or financial, and is a violation by a person who has power over the life of a vulnerable adult. Different types of abuse range from physical abuse such as assault, to psychological abuse, including deprivation of contact, control, intimidation, financial abuse, neglect and acts of omission, and discriminatory behaviour.

The aim of this chapter is twofold: to begin to lift the veil from this uncomfortable subject, and to challenge some of the assumptions that underpin beliefs surrounding it. We seek to identify and illustrate three distinctive types of abuse in the palliative care context: **established abuse, institutional abuse**, and **unwitting abuse.** These concepts will be developed in relation to children and families, vulnerable adults, staff behaviour and the treatment of staff, past trauma, and bereavement, and finally relocated within the context of human rights. By attempting to raise the profile of abuse in its many and diverse guises, our intention is to stimulate debate about abuse and the care of dying people. Arising out of this discussion will be indicators for practice. We note that little appears to have been written so far about abuse in palliative care, but hope that this contribution may be the basis of future work.

When considering what we have called **established abuse**, we are attempting to describe a situation where the abusive relationships or behaviour pre-date the palliative care contact. The prevalence of various forms of violence in families, and the pressure to keep silent in the past, means that those who care for the dying are often witnesses to behaviour, conversations, and symptoms of past trauma and abuse, as well as ongoing demeaning and abusive relationships. In our practice we have observed many different permutations of ongoing and established abuse when a family member is dying and have seen these pre-existing coping styles and patterns of behaviour exacerbated or exposed by the crisis of a terminal illness. In our practice we have supported: women carers who are belittled and shouted at by the patient at visiting time; a mother in physical danger of assault from her dying and mentally ill son; an elderly, incontinent alcoholic father living in squalor with his son, who is also drinking heavily; situations where the abuser has been either the patient (perhaps a husband 'heavy with his fists'), or a carer (aggressive to visiting care staff, and demanding the patient to continue to behave as if they were well). In many instances, established patterns of behaviour may be very difficult to challenge, and particular forms of behaviour may stretch back over generations.

In the context of working with the dying, where time frames are limited by the progression of a patient's disease, the challenge for workers lies in arriving at some kind of judgement as to what can or should be changed and challenged. How realistic is it to expect an elderly person to change the way they speak of and treat their partner, or female staff, or their self-abuse? Do victims want to challenge or change their situation, when it may come to an end by death anyway? The main thrust of the palliative care worker may be simply to be aware of the issues, to have our assumptions challenged about how families work, and to try to protect other people from the effects of the abuse.

We have used the term **institutional abuse** to describe a situation where the key factors include equity of access to services, the use and prioritization of scarce resources, discrimination, power in staff teams, and the treatment and behaviour of staff. This is often a difficult area for palliative care as it confronts the 'culture of niceness' (Gunaratnam 2000) so prevalent in hospice settings. Gunaratnam identifies the difficulties that palliative care staff have in debating and addressing institutional racism, and we would suggest this applies to all forms of institutional abuse. This is due in part to the implicit challenge to their public persona of goodness and compassion, where staff are 'valued for their heroic abilities to nurture and to provide universal care for vulnerable individuals' (Gunaratnam 2000). Palliative care staff find it difficult to contemplate that there may be issues to raise about the safety and practice of their colleagues, or how colleagues treat each other in the work-place, as it would fracture the image of the palliative care worker as one who 'has a vocational calling' to work with dying people (Gunaratnam 2000). Gunaratnam suggests that institutional racism (and, we believe, by extension, other forms of institutional abuse) is generated within the specific dynamics of palliative care due to the founding history, 'structures, philosophies and practices within the speciality' in the way in which palliative care prides itself on individualized care for each unique person as they are dying. This means that palliative care workers can avoid addressing wider social inequalities such as racism, poverty, or abuses of power, by both professional and family carers, as not being relevant to the care of any individual patient and family.

Unwitting abuse occurs when a person could be seen to be abusive, even though acting with the best of intentions. In these situations there is often a conflict of values or rights, and whether the outcome is interpreted as abusive is open to question. Unwitting abuse can often arise when assumptions are made about others, and actions taken, without being checked. This can give rise to the danger of projecting our own values and concerns onto other people, assuming that they are shared. There are no clear definitions or absolutes about unwitting abuse, but rather a contested exercise of power, and the palliative care worker or family member may be an abuser in this situation in their attempt to reduce or manage risk.

For example, a middle-aged woman with Down's syndrome, moderate learning difficulties, and some physical disability lived with her elderly parents. When she was diagnosed with cancer, her parents refused to consider her wish to return to her adult training centre, or 'school' as the family called it, or to see her 'school friends'. Despite her repeated requests to see friends, and her wishes for a different lifestyle, her physical dependency meant that she did not realize these hopes. Her parents feared that she would be upset, unsafe, and could be taken ill. Instead she was laid on the sofa at home, her favourite foods brought to her, and she died, beautifully cared for, without ever leaving the house again. Motivated by fear and love, and despite all attempts to reassure them, the parents felt a huge sense of parental and moral responsibility to keep their daughter with them and provide her with good quality care. Her parents would be horrified if this was construed as abuse, and certainly did not intend to abuse her. However, their actions did deprive their daughter of her choice and the autonomy to which she was entitled as an adult during the final months of her life.

Laudable motivation, rights, responsibilities, differing values within different professions, and different perceptions of risk when caring for the dying often bring us into conflict, when trying to provide the best quality of care.

Vulnerable adults and abuse

The recognition and awareness of the vulnerability of adults and the need for thought about their protection has slowly developed in Britain, starting with medical observation of 'granny battering', in the mid 1970s, to the consequent development by social service departments of local policies and procedures over the past twenty years. There is no criminal offence of neglecting a dependent adult of sound mind (although they are afforded legal protection if they are living in residential or nursing care), and there is no statutory duty for children to care for their parents, unlike in some other European countries. Some physical acts against vulnerable adults, such as assault or financial abuse are criminally punishable. Omissions are harder to criminalize. It is in this legal context that most local authorities have developed policies to protect adults with learning difficulties and elderly people from abuse, and most have multi-agency protocols for vulnerable adults in place. By placing expectations on workers to be 'alerters' to abuse, employers have also had to produce other policies and procedures regarding harassment at work and whistle blowing.

In palliative care in the UK, the requirements of the Care Standards Act (2000) require hospices, in particular, to consider their policies regarding whistle-blowing, dignity at work, and child and adult protection, and many palliative care units are having to consider these organizational issues of established and institutional abuse for the first time.

Often the response to producing these policies in palliative care is one of distancing: 'we don't need that type of thing here', 'it is politically correct nonsense', or 'love for one another is enough, we are all here to do the best for our patients'. These policies do however, flow from a respect for the rights of vulnerable adults and aspire actively to promote the empowerment and well being of vulnerable patients, whilst also recognizing that the right to self-determination can involve risk. These ought to be familiar and shared aspirations in palliative care.

Skinner (1998) identified three roles within adult protection: alerting, investigating, and managing. Palliative care staff will usually be required to be alerters only. They are rarely asked to verify or prove that information is true, but rather to log concerns and report them to the appropriate authorities. This is the first step in the process of keeping people safe and empowering them for the future. However, to be an effective alerter, one also has to be alert to recognizing the signs of adult abuse, to recognizing bad practice, and to know how and whom to alert.

A complication in considering abuse in the context of palliative care is that many of the indicators of adult abuse will arise during the course of a final illness, and may not be an indicator of abusive behaviour but rather the symptoms of the dying trajectory. For example, lack of appetite, high levels of anxiety, changed personal appearance, unexpected shifts in mood and behaviour, sleep disturbance, emotional flatness and withdrawal, are all possible indicators of abuse, but could also be observed in people who have secondary brain cancer, who are toxic, or who are appropriately sad or anxious as their life comes to an end. This has certainly prevented some palliative care teams from adopting polices which they feel do not accurately express the particular and specialized situation of the dying. However, perhaps a more appropriate response would be to consider that abuse can occur in any setting, no matter where the person lives or who is caring for them, and to bear to contemplate this disturbing possibility, to make a skilled assessment, and to have some knowledge of pre-disposing factors which may lead to abuse.

In the domestic setting, where there is what we have described as long established abuse, these predisposing factors may include situations where for years family relationships have been poor and where family violence is the norm. A large amount of elder abuse is ongoing domestic violence, where abuse of alcohol or drugs are often key factors. Carer stresses are significant, such as carers feeling unsupported and isolated, and where they have unwillingly had to change their lifestyle, or where the carer is being abused or subject to excessive demands from the ill person. For example, an elderly man, with end-stage pulmonary disease, insisted that his wife slept sitting in a chair at his bedside. As soon as her only remaining supportive friend visited, he would make enormous demands to disrupt the visit, and refused to allow any professional carers over the threshold to the point where his wife described their relationship in these words, 'he used to be my soul-mate and now he's my cell-mate'.

The research of Homer and Gilleard (1990), however, challenges the stereotypical image of the over-stressed daughter of the heavily dependent elderly person being driven to abuse by stress. They found that it is more important to consider the characteristics of the abuser, and that, for example, alcohol consumption was a significant factor and verbally abusive behaviour was often long-standing. Perpetrators of abuse in the home have been found to have a high incidence of arrest, hospitalization for psychiatric conditions, or have limited functioning due to their own health problems. A perpetrator is often emotionally dependent on the elderly person they victimize, and 'the abuse appears to be a reflection of the perpetrator's problems and dependency, rather than the elderly victim's characteristics' (Wiehe 1998). This dependency and these conflicted relationships can have implications for the bereavement care of those who are mourning a spouse or parent who has abused them.

Abuse in palliative care is experienced in many different configurations. An illustration from our practice is the large number issues raised when an abusive father was dying. These included how he related to his daughters that he had sexually abused as children, (who were now also his carers), his abuse and harassment of nursing staff even as he was dying, the daughters' concern for his care, but also their distress at their past experiences, and their anger with a mother who had not protected them. Further complications included the feelings of the staff towards the patient, the management of his behaviour towards them, the bereavement needs of the daughters and wife, and the secrecy, which cloaked it all. This led staff to make judgements about family functioning, and power relationships in the family. They felt anger towards the wife, who they assumed had condoned or tolerated her husband's behaviour and not protected her daughters, and this was compounded by the nurses' distaste and anger at the patient's continuing sexual harassment and their own vulnerability. Secrecy, as in this case, is often threatened by impending loss, which can be a trigger factor of abusive memories (Hunt et al. 1997).

The abuse of vulnerable adults can be subtle, is not necessarily violent, and is often about previous difficult social relationships, issues of power, and competing needs. In palliative care the practice issues include: a willingness to consider that abuse may be an issue; to learn about pre-disposing factors and indicators; and to realize that empowerment of vulnerable adults is crucial, as victims' wishes are paramount, and intervention is usually only possible with their agreement. The issue is one of self-determination and human rights, not of rescuing the victim. Adoption of inter-agency policies and procedures, and being willing to contemplate being an alerter is a start, for the prospect of alerting others to abuse can be daunting, especially where the alerter has been the only one to suspect or witness the abuse. By affirming our personal values and being careful not to project our personal memories or experience of abuse on to colleagues, patients, or carers, we can maintain our personal and professional integrity and avoid abusing others.

A different type of abuse, which is quite regularly observed by palliative care practitioners, is the behaviour and distress of dying people whose earlier lives include traumatic experience of war, persecution, refugee experiences, sexual and family violence. For example, caring for people who have been prisoners of war in the Far East, when their awareness of impending death seems to trigger a sudden upsurge of old traumatic memories, distress, and emotional pain. Crocq (1997) comments that current losses, such as loss of career, status, illness, and increasing dependency may re-invoke a sense of the helplessness and powerlessness previously experienced, and patients are no longer able to suppress these memories. Dying is a time of life review and preparation for endings, but these memories may be very vivid and distressing. Crocq (1997) describes the intrusive nature of traumatic recollections, the painful and abnormally high levels of psychological and physical anxiety, the often obsessive thought processes about shocking wartime events, guilt, and the surprise of the patients at the firm entrenchment of these memories with their continuing power to hurt. Another factor may be the difficulty family members have in observing the outbreak of what often has been previously a silent and suppressed pain.

Children and abuse

People may talk about childhood abuse and failed relationships as they are dying, but palliative care staff also have an obligation to consider the young users – patients, bereaved children, or visitors of their services today, and to have appropriate procedures and policies in place. Increasing legislation regarding statutory checks on all staff working with children, and risk assessments for children visiting a hospice or attending a group for bereaved children has made palliative care units realize that our 'culture of niceness' is not enough.

Abuse of children in a palliative care setting may take many different forms and degrees of severity, such as: the long established abuse of a child being mistreated or neglected by a family member; the unwitting abuse of over-protection from bad news, which so often disables and distresses children for years to come; the institutional abuse of not planning for the needs of children and young people as visitors or service users. Many units have established policies and procedures, which arise from taking the human rights of children seriously. For example the Sue Ryder Care Child Protection Policy and Procedures states that a child needs to 'be valued as an individual, to be treated with dignity and respect, to be cared for as a child first, to be safe' (Sue Ryder Care 2003). This in turn requires palliative care workers to consider how they work with young carers and the appropriateness of burdens placed on them. Other practice indicators may include considering disabled access to services provided for children, the design and content of information for children and young people with a learning disability, as well as the responsibility on staff as possible 'alerters', to have knowledge and understanding of local child protection procedures and how to act on concerns and disclosures.

Staff and abuse

Staff in palliative care settings can be abusers, and the registration and inspection of all type of palliative care services, as well as whistle blowing polices, are an attempt to deal with the abuse of vulnerable dying or bereaved people by staff. We all have the potential to be unwitting abusers, because we all bring personal biographies to our work, which include our professional value systems, our own experiences of abuse and family life, our expectations about what families should do and what is acceptable behaviour. Whilst we might all share core values such as patients' rights and autonomy, utility, justice, compassion, and whole person care (Randal and Downie 1996), the interpretation of these values will inevitably differ between individuals. Power relationships within multi-disciplinary teams (Hugman 1986) will also influence the degree to which different staff have access to the debate. The debate might be about: risk-taking, the extent of the responsibility of carers, who should get a service, or the care of the unpopular patient. An insight into our own agendas and values helps us to be alert to our own potential for unwitting abuse.

Staff may also experience abuse from colleagues and managers, through racism or ageism in the work place, as well as abuse from users of the service. Abuse in the workplace can take the form of bullying, harassment, or disparagement and scapegoating, as well as oppression and discrimination. There may be sexual harassment, victimization of whistle-blowers, exploitation of the workforce, or a failure to support front-line staff adequately. 'The degree of intentionality varies; some perpetrators may be partially unaware of their actions, or an abusive outcome may result from a series of neglectful or incompetent decisions. ... There is little consensus about what is unlawful, unethical, unacceptable and what is merely trivial and irritating' (Brearley 2000). When working with the dying there are perhaps particular difficulties in addressing institutional abuse. The historical development and underlying ethos of the palliative care movement with its 'charismatic leadership, narrow focus, Christian ethos, and highly committed and socially homogeneous group of founder members' (James N, Field D in Gunaratnam 2000), has meant that these issues are only slowly being addressed. There is sometimes pressure on staff to do more than is reasonable, to 'donate' extra time, to work for lower rates of pay, to tolerate poor working conditions, to accept a relentless workload, and staff often collude with this because they are working with dying people, or for a charity, and tomorrow will be too late.

Racism in the workplace is the day-to-day experience for many nursing and medical staff. Following the Stephen Lawrence Inquiry (MacPherson 1999), addressing institutional racism in palliative care should be seen as a priority. Racist abuse from patients to other service users or towards staff is something many palliative care workers find difficult to deal with in a setting that has tended to emphasize 'cultural sensitivity rather than race equality' (Gunaratnam 2000). There is a sense of futility and discomfort in confronting the behaviour of people who are elderly and dying. This is discussed in Gunaratnam's research that considers the dilemma of nursing staff about how, and when it is appropriate to challenge racism by service users (Gunaratnam 2001). She views palliative care as a ground-breaking movement that now needs to turn its attention to its own policies, procedures, education, and training, and develop an organizational culture that empowers staff to speak out. Addressing the issues of abuse in the workplace, Brearley highlights some practice indicators: the adequate provision of human relations training and support for managers, stress awareness input at all levels, and human resources policy documents stating values, rules, and clear guidance on procedures, made credible by firm implementation when required (Brearley in McCluskey and Hooper 2000).

Bereavement and abuse

There is an enormous literature on bereavement, grief, grief counselling, and grief therapy, and setting up and running bereavement support services in all their various forms. For practitioners, abuse and bereavement is an important topic in two main areas. Firstly to design a bereavement care service that is not institutionally abusive to vulnerable grieving people. Secondly to help us understand how bereaved people who have been in established abusive relationships may cope with their loss. When considering offering bereavement care, an organization needs to be aware of the potential for being 'institutionally abusive', and to consider such issues as access to its services, the timing of events, the recruitment, and training of supporters/counsellors representing a cross section of the community that is supported, as well as the often thorny issue of the religious content of any act of remembrance.

People make themselves vulnerable when they seek support for their distress and grief, so there are also important issues to consider regarding their safety if they are being visited in their own home. Organizations have a responsibility for the vetting and training of bereavement visitors. Sadly, financial abuse of vulnerable people at a time of great turmoil and change is not unknown. Another area to consider is the support of volunteer staff in helping them set appropriate boundaries when working with bereaved people. The aim is to help them avoid situations where the isolated or lonely person wants the counselling relationship to become an ongoing friendship or something more intimate.

Unwitting abuse may arise in bereavement support if we make assumptions, and then judgements, about the lifestyle, values, and relationships that people have had, and the way we think that they ought to react to bereavement. How do our values about family life, respect, appropriate length of mourning, affect our support for the young widower who starts a new relationship within a few months of his wife's death?

Bereaved people who have experienced abuse have been identified as at high risk of complicated grief, as they often have had a highly ambivalent relationship with their abuser and this 'usually portends excessive amounts of anger and guilt which causes the survivor difficulty' (Worden 1991). There is a considerable psychiatric literature on the difficulties of ending relationships that have been a mixture of love and hate, where ambivalence is identified as a cause of intense and prolonged mourning. The death of a family member, with the breaking of family secrets and myths that may accompany it, can also throw a whole family into crisis and disequilibrium. It is important to consider the whole family system when unresolved or complicated grief is present as 'it may not only serve as a key factor in family pathology but may contribute to pathological relationships across the generations' (Worden 1991). In this way established abuse within the family may cast a long shadow, and practitioners need to consider whether abuse is a significant factor when supporting bereaved people.

Human rights and abuse

If abuse in palliative care is to be tackled effectively it is vital for staff to have a working knowledge of any legislation that exists to enable this. In the UK this would include an understanding of the Children Act 1989, Race Relations Act 2000, and Carers and Disability Discrimination Acts 1995. In addition, each professional group should be familiar with their own codes of practice/ethics relating to their work. For example, in the UK, the General Social Care Council's comprehensive code for social workers and social care workers includes requirements for workers to ensure the protection and uphold the rights and interests of service users and carers, and an obligation to ensure that their behaviour does not harm themselves or other people. The code also specifies the need for 'relevant colleagues and agencies to be informed about the outcomes and implications of risk assessments' (GSCC 2000). In order for palliative care staff to become more effective 'alerters' they need to feel confident in their own knowledge base, understand their professional obligations and, in particular, to feel supported by their employers.

The Human Rights Act 1998 brings all existing law under the umbrella of European legislation making it possible for cases to be pursued in the British Courts, and British legislation must be interpreted in relation to the convention rights. There are sixteen basic rights covering all aspects of life, including the right to life itself, as well as property, marriage, family life, education, and freedom of expression.

Case Law is now beginning to emerge, and at a time when there are ongoing debates on assisted suicide and euthanasia, the right to life under Article 2 has received much publicity. In a recent landmark case in the UK, Diane Pretty, who suffered from advanced motor neurone disease, requested immunity from prosecution for her husband, who she wished to assist her to commit suicide. She asserted that her quality of life constituted inhuman and degrading treatment in contravention of Article 3. This case demonstrates the problems inherent in the Act where convention rights may conflict. In this instance the judges felt that the right to life, (Article 2), took precedence over Mrs Pretty's perception of her palliative care as 'inhumane and degrading treatment', and she lost her case, dying of her disease some weeks later.

Jane and Peter illustrate a less obvious example, where both parties had a moral case for protection under the Act. Jane had a rare and fluctuating terminal condition, which meant that her estranged husband returned to the marital home to care for their two sons during a period of respite care. When Jane was ready for discharge Peter asserted a right to the property as a means of ensuring continuity and a stable base for their sons. Article 8 of the Human Rights Act confers the right to respect for private and family life, home and correspondence, and Article 1 of Protocol 1, the peaceful right to the enjoyment of one's possessions. In theory, these rights should apply equally to both parties. In the event, however, Jane was left effectively homeless, the last year of her life was spent in a hospice, and then a nursing home, unable to enjoy her own possessions or family life. Had the Act been invoked on her behalf, it would have been difficult to predict the outcome.

Although the Human Rights Act identifies clear parameters in relation to all major aspects of life, the key to its effectiveness as a means of preventing abuse lies in the establishment of case law. As lawyers continue to interpret the Act, its effects will become clearer. Despite a suggestion that initial implementation has been cautious, less radical, and accessed only by the rich and famous, the Human Rights Act is important and will inform future practice. In the context of palliative care, 'it can be the trigger that promotes greater attention to adult protection issues.' (Valios 2003)

Indicators for practice

Arising from this general overview of abuse in palliative care, we suggest the following practice indicators may be useful:

◆ The introduction of comprehensive policies and protocols on abuse in all specialist palliative care settings

◆ The inclusion of abuse and human rights training in formal education programmes for palliative care staff

◆ The proactive fostering of a culture in the workplace which encourages openness in relation to issues of abuse

◆ Awareness that leads to considering the possibility of abuse as an integral part of risk assessment

◆ All information should be available in a range of formats, to ensure that it is accessible to all user groups.

Conclusion

In a specialty that is primarily concerned with death and dying it is hardly surprising that we should need to emphasize the more positive aspects of our work as a means of self-preservation. However, if significant progress is to be made it has to be acknowledged that abuse occurs and is everybody's business. As general awareness about human rights grows, palliative care staff need to engage with this debate and can no longer afford to evade this topic. Openness and awareness provide the key to challenging the abuse of power that is the common denominator in all forms of abuse.

References

Brearley J (2000) Working as an organizational consultant with abuse encountered in the workplace. In McCluskey U and Hooper C (ed.) *Psychodynamic Perspectives on Abuse: The Cost of Fear*, pp 223–43. Jessica Kingsley Publishers, London.

Crocq L (1997) The emotional consequences of war 50 years on. A psychiatrist's perspective. In Hunt l, Marshall M, and Rowlings C (ed.) *Past Trauma in Late Life European Perspectives on Therapeutic Work with Older People*, pp. 39–49. Jessica Kingsley Publishers, London.

Gunaratnam Y (2000) Implications of the Stephen Lawrence inquiry for palliative care. *International Journal of Palliative Nursing* 6(3):147–9.

Gunaratnam Y (2001) "We mustn't judge people… but": staff dilemmas in dealing with racial harassment amongst hospice service users. *Sociology of Health and Illness* 23(1):65–84.

GSCC (2002) *Codes of Practice for Social Care Workers and Employers*. General Social Care Council, London.

Homer A and Gilleard C (1990) Abuse of elderly people by their carers. *British Medical Journal* 301:1359-62.

Hugman R (1986) *Power in Helping Professions*. Macmillan Press, London.

Human Rights Act 1998: Study Guide (2000) Home Office Communication Directorate, London.

Hunt L, Marshall M, and Rowlings C (1997) *Past Trauma in Late Life: European Perspectives on Therapeutic Work with Older People*. Jessica Kingsley Publishers, London.

McCluskey U and Hooper C (2000) (ed.) *Psychodynamic Perspectives on Abuse: The Cost of Fear*. Jessica Kingsley Publishers, London.

MacPherson W (1999) *The Stephen Lawrence Inquiry: Report of an Inquiry by Sir William MacPherson of Cluny*. Home Office, London.

Randal F and Downie R (1996) *Palliative Care Ethics. A Good Companion*. Oxford Medical Publications, Oxford.

Skinner B *et al.* (1998) *AIMS for Adult Protection – The Alerter's Guide*. Pavilion Publishing, Brighton.

Valios N (2003) Time to read the Rights Act, *Community Care*, 23/29 Jan, pp. 30–31.

Wiehe V (1998) *Understanding Family Violence*. Sage Publications Inc, California.

Sue Ryder Care (2003) *Child Protection Policies and Procedures*. Manorlands Sue Ryder Care.

Worden WJ (1991) *Grief Counselling and Grief Therapy*. Routledge, London.

9

Offenders

Maggie Bolger

Introduction

Individuals who come into prison are socially excluded from the general population. However, as members of a democratic society, we have a duty to provide for their health and social care needs. This chapter will explore a number of challenging issues including the nature and purpose of imprisonment; the health and social needs of prisoners, as well as the losses that have to be endured by an individual coming into the prison system. The second half of the chapter will focus upon the losses that an individual with a life threatening condition may experience. I will examine some of the coping mechanisms that are often adopted in order to deal with the losses imposed by both the illness and incarceration. In particular, Worden's four tasks of grieving will be discussed and adapted to assist carers in supporting and assisting prisoners, who are also individuals in need, in coming to terms with loss within the secure environment. The final part of this chapter will look at recent innovations in prison health care, as well as offering guidance in relation to the development of palliative care services for prisoners.

The nature and purpose of imprisonment

What purpose does a term of imprisonment serve? What can we as members of a democratic society expect of it? What effect does incarceration have upon an individual?

To many, the subject matter of prison, imprisonment, and prisoners is very emotive. On a regular basis newspapers report rising levels of crime, most of which appear to be of a violent nature. Some individuals appear to regard prison as a 'soft option' that does not seem to do much in reducing the rates of recidivism. Public opinion is often influenced by media reports of high-profile offenders and the crimes that they have committed. As a consequence, some may find it difficult to feel compassion or sympathy for the rapist, paedophile, or murderer who becomes seriously ill whilst in prison. It may seem easier to empathize with an individual who develops a serious illness if they are convicted of a minor crime, or where they are known to have come from a disadvantaged background.

In order to answer the above questions, Coyle (2001) suggests that it is useful to differentiate between what is meant by the **act** of imprisonment, and the **experience** of imprisonment. Coyle explains that the act of imprisonment is carried out by the magistrate or judge who deems that the individual has committed a crime that determines that he/she should be deprived of their liberty. In sentencing, the judge will have taken into account the seriousness of the crime, as well as public sentiment concerning the nature of the crime committed. For those entering prison, especially for the first time, they find the prison environment a strange, hostile, and uncertain world, where fears over personal safety and loss of family ties are examples of some of the many losses that are to be endured by the individual. We must remember that individuals enter prison as *part* of their punishment, and *not for* punishment. Removal of liberty for a defined period of time, along with attempts to rehabilitate the individual is the guiding principle behind imprisonment.

The United Kingdom Prison Service Mission states that:
'Her Majesty's Prison Service serves the public by keeping in custody those committed by the courts. Our duty is to look after them with humanity and help them lead law-abiding and useful lives in custody and on release.'

The prison experience should be a positive one, one that facilitates the individual to address their offending behaviour in a humane way, as well as learn new work and life skills that will enable them to lead more law-abiding lives whilst in custody and then on release.

The prison population

The prison population in the United Kingdom currently stands at around 73,000 individuals. The vast majority of offenders are male between the ages of 15 and 80 years of age. Prisons in the United Kingdom are overcrowded and have been for the past 20 years. Newell (2003) cites Train (1991) that the problems of overcrowding have a negative effect upon the life and work of prisons, which in turn produce intolerable conditions for both prisoners and staff alike. Overcrowding 'cripples' the ability of the prison system to deliver programmes and treatment in a timely and appropriate manner; overcrowding diverts resources away from those who might benefit from them, as well as increasing stress and potential danger for staff and prisoners (Newell 2003). It is not difficult to appreciate that providing equitable health care within such an environment is likely to be extremely challenging.

The health and social needs of prisoners

It is acknowledged that prisoners are a transient population, who generally spend only a short amount of time in prison before returning to the wider community. However, many take with them their health and social care needs (DOH 1999). The general health care of prisoners has been the subject of debate over the last few years (BMA 1996; Smith 1997). The British Medical Association, as long ago as 1993, pointed out that prisoners were less healthy and had greater medical needs than that of the general population (BMA 1993). In 1997, Reed and Lyne carried out a series of inspections and found that in 10 of the 19 prisons studied in England and Wales the standard of health care received by prisoners was variable, and in many instances was of 'low quality'.

However, it was not until 1999, following a number of reports and inspections related to the prison estate (e.g. *'Patient or Prisoner'* 1996) that *The Future Organisation of Prison Health Care* published by the Joint Prison Service/National Health Service Executive Working Group (DOH 1999) finally acknowledged that health care was inconsistent in British prisons and that in some instances it fell below the standard that was provided in the wider community. The report followed an investigation into conditions at Wormwood Scrubs (1999) where concerns in relation to the provision of health care were identified. The report drew attention to the fact that it was the 'most unwell and vulnerable' prisoners who received the 'worst regime.'

Individuals in prison will present with a diverse range of health and social care needs that may present significant challenges to staff on a day-to-day basis in relation to 'care verses custody' issues (BMA 1993; Fursland 1999; U.K.C.C. 1999). The predominant concerns are those related to mental health problems (both acute and long standing), substance misuse, as well as a number of physical health needs, such as respiratory diseases, oral health problems, as well as chronic health problems such as coronary heart disease, cancers, arthritis, multiple sclerosis.

In the United States there has been a 50% rise in the number of older prisoners since 1996. Lemieux *et al.* (2002) describe this growth as unprecedented and one that is leading policy makers to review a number of important issues, such as the economic costs of holding individuals in prison for long periods of time, the cost to the state of providing specialized health care, as compared to the concerns for public safety, institutional management, and humanitarian concerns. In their review of the literature, they found that 83% of older U.S. prisoners had at least one chronic health problem, and that 49% had three or more. Prisoners who were segregated had greater demands for health care than those who were not. Older prisoners experiencing ill health and age-related losses were most likely to report symptoms of depression and anxiety. The possibility of dying in prison was a predominant fear expressed to the staff that cared for them. The United Kingdom has an ageing population. As the prison population continues to rise, it is likely that the number of ageing prisoners will also increase. If this occurs, then it is possible that we may also see a rise in the number of chronic medical conditions, requiring palliative interventions, such as pain and symptom management. In the future, it is likely that British policy makers will also have to consider the same issues as counterparts in the United States.

In the general population, individuals who have both chronic and enduring health and social care needs are usually able to access specialist care services and teams. However, for the individual who is also a prisoner this is not as easy. For example, the need to ensure security may conflict with the need to provide appropriate health and social care for this socially excluded, but vulnerable group of individuals.

The primary concern of a prison is to ensure the protection of the public from individuals deemed to be a risk to society because of their criminal behaviour. Prisons are not sufficiently resourced to cater for the diverse range of health and social care needs of their population in the longer term. Prison Governors are often faced with a number of difficult decisions to make when allocating scarce budgetary resources across a range of prison activities, such as maintaining security, providing purposeful activity for prisoners, as well as catering for their immediate health and social care needs.

Many prisons in the United Kingdom do not have health facilities that are appropriately staffed and commensurate with the National Health Service. This is something that the Government recognizes and is attempting to address. However, in the meantime, an ever increasing prison population, prisoner classification, as well as the need to conform to the prison system as a whole can frustrate plans of care. Such constraints may mean that the opportunities to treat prisoners as individuals, as well as involvement of the family in times of chronic illness are diminished.

For many individuals, coming into prison may provide their first contact with health and social care services for a number of years. Some may not even be registered with a community doctor (General Practitioner). Individuals are often in a poor state of health, both physically and mentally on arrival. It is possible that a medical problem, such as cancer, may have gone undetected for some time and this may mean that palliation of symptoms is all that can be realistically achieved.

The World Health Organisation (1998) emphasizes that the loss of liberty constitutes punishment, and that the health and well being of an individual in prison must not to be compromised. Prison has the potential to make a difference. The prison population represents some of the most vulnerable in our society who have multiple and unmet health needs. Good health and social care in prisons would benefit the individual as well as the community, and this may in turn reduce rates of re-offending. Better health and social care received whilst in prison may also help prevent acute breakdown and tragic incidents such as suicide and murders committed by people with mental health problems (DOH 1999; McManus 2001).

Prison health care in the United Kingdom is undergoing a period of dramatic change, and as such provides dynamic opportunities for the development of palliative care services within this, the most challenging of health care environments. *The Future Organisation of Prison Health Care* (1999) asserted that better health care could be found in prisons that had good partnerships with local health providers. In April 2003, the funding of prison health care transferred from the Prison Service to the government Department of Health. This is an important step forward in the development of equitable standards of healthcare. However, it is pertinent to note that the British Medical Association report (2001) *Prison Medicine: A crisis waiting to break,* pinpointed the scarcity of resources, both human and financial, and recommended that the Government should recognize the need for greater financial support to prison health services. Taking prison health initiatives forward is likely to present a number of additional challenges for a National Health Service whose resources are scarce. It is unlikely that the general public will support costly health interventions that take place within the confines of a prison.

Prison, an environment of enduring loss?

Any individual entering a prison will find that they have to cope with a number of losses, which are likely to result in expressions of grief and bereavement. There are the obvious losses: loss of liberty; loss of family ties; loss of income and employment etc. However, there are many other losses, actual and perceived, that may not be so readily apparent. These losses include:

- Liberty
- Family ties
- Heterosexual relationships
- Income/employment
- Life years
- Privacy
- Shame and stigma, associated with incarceration
- Physical and social space
- Time, especially individual structure to the day
- Individual roles, such as husband, wife, employee etc
- Human contact and acceptance
- Personal safety and security
- Personal autonomy
- Personal possessions
- Decision making and feeling in control of their situation
- Forms of communication, such as telephones etc
- Freedom of speech and expression
- Cultural and religious diversification

Individual coping and adaptation mechanisms

Although each individual will vary in their personal response to the losses imposed upon them by coming into prison, Matthews (1999) has identified three general modes of adaptation, as outlined below:

1. *Co-operation or colonization*—the individual prisoner will aim to keep out of trouble and do their time with minimal conflict and stress. The aim is to work towards reaching their earliest release dates;

2. *Withdrawal*—The individual may choose to withdraw physically and socially from other prisoners. The individual may also self-harm, attempt suicide, as well as exhibiting signs of depression;

3. *Rebellion and resistance*—this may either involve various forms of non-cooperation at one extreme to disturbances and riots at the other.

Death, dying, and coping within prison

We have so far explored the effect that prison has upon an individual and identified the possible coping mechanisms that may be adopted. However, when an individual in prison has a life threatening condition, how does he/she cope? Is the prison a suitable environment in which to be cared for, or in which to die? What effect does the prison environment have on the coping mechanisms of the dying prisoner?

In order to answer these questions, we should first remind ourselves of the core principles of palliative care, as identified by Faull *et al.* (1998):

♦ Achievement of the best quality of life for patients and their families

♦ Good control of symptoms

♦ Facilitate adjustment of losses and 'unfinished business'

♦ A dignified death, with minimal distress, in the patient's own place of choosing

♦ Prevention of problems in bereavement.

If it is possible, a prison will apply to the Home Secretary to grant release on compassionate grounds. The individual will then hopefully be able die peacefully at home or in the local hospice. However, obtaining release on compassionate grounds can take time to achieve, and may not be feasible for certain prisoners, depending on the nature of their criminal offence, e.g. drug trafficking, or where an individual has a severe personality disorder that may make them a significant risk to the public if released. Such an individual is therefore likely to die inside the prison.

Many prisoners will view death in prison as the ultimate failure, and it is not difficult to see why. One of the basic privileges each of us would request is the right to die, with dignity and peace, in a place of our own choosing, surrounded by family and friends. How many would want to die in a secure environment, where simple gestures such as touch may be frowned upon, without family and friends at our side, and where the opportunities to discuss the dying process and make decisions about care may be limited?

Currently, in order to care appropriately for individuals in prison, with a life-threatening condition, there are a number of challenges that will need to be overcome in order to fulfil the core principles described by Faull *et al.* above. Briefly, these can be identified as the:

♦ conformity that prisons have to adopt to the rules and regulations, rather than having the flexibility to allow for individual choice;

◆ problems of overcrowding and poor facilities in some prisons may diminish opportunities to treat prisoners as individuals and to involve their families;

◆ concerns about drug abuse may restrain efforts to provide appropriate pain and symptom control. In addition, pain relief using opiate drugs may also be difficult to achieve because of concerns over drug abuse. A lack of knowledge in the prison staff of pain and symptom management can leave them feeling isolated. This isolation may be further exacerbated when outside agencies, such as primary health care trusts, are reluctant to engage in joint service provision;

◆ overall communication and delivery of service are complicated by the need to ensure security and public protection.

The United States prison hospice movement

In the United States hospice care for prisoners is now well established in a number of states. It developed out of the need to provide palliative care for an increasing number of prisoners diagnosed as HIV positive in the mid-1980s. In the United States, longer sentences, limited use of parole and compassionate release, has meant that death in prison is now a reality for many prisoners. The United States Prison Hospice Association was established in the mid-1990s, and in 1998 standards of practice were developed out of the GRACE Project—'Guiding Responsive Action for Corrections in End of Life'.

The GRACE Project was initiated to increase knowledge about end of life care. It started out by trying to identify what end of life programmes were currently taking place in prisons and jails across the country. Two of the most challenging issues reported related to pain and symptom management (similar to that described above for UK prisons), and family visitation and involvement. The distance and estrangement from family and difficulty in arranging and extending out of hours visits meant that family ties were either lost or strained (Ratcliff 2002).

The GRACE Project therefore sought to create and promote quality end of life programmes that could be implemented across the country. One of the most innovative aspects of these care programmes concerned the involvement of other prisoners as hospice volunteers, 'as no one understands a prisoner like another prisoner.'

In an earlier article, Ratcliff (2000) drew attention to the fact that a death in custody was often equated with neglect, and raised potential legal, ethical, and medical complications. She reported that prisoners were often expected to go to hospital 'in shackles' to die. For many seriously ill prisoners, who had been incarcerated for many years, or who had become alienated from family and friends, prison had become their 'home'. Therefore, the use of Advance Directives, including 'Do Not Attempt Resuscitation' orders allowed the prisoner to die with dignity in prison, rather than be moved to a hospital to die 'in shackles'. It could be argued that the use of such directives allowed the prisoner some degree of choice and flexibility regarding their place of death.

Assisting individuals to adjust to life-threatening conditions in prison

Tillman (2000) describes, based on the experience of the United States, the psychological needs of the terminally ill:

◆ *A feeling of security*—as the prisoner begins to do less for himself, fear over personal safety becomes more of an issue. He is at risk from others of violence and manipulation from other prisoners.

◆ *To feel needed and not a burden*—the prisoner may more readily accept help from another prisoner than he will from staff or family members.

◆ *Explanation of symptoms and nature of the disease*—prison dehumanises an individual. The perception may be that they require less explanation/information than those in the 'free world'

◆ *Human contact and acceptance*—simple gesture, such as touch may be discouraged in the prison environment, for fear of misinterpretation or manipulation by the prisoner.

◆ *Opportunities to discuss the process of dying*—individuals may perceive that their status as prisoners leads to sub-standard care and treatment.

◆ *Involvement in decision-making and honest communication*—how an individual dies requires advance care planning. The prospect of making such decisions may prove overwhelming to some. The prisoner may see some staff as untrustworthy. Prison volunteers can act as effective mediators between the seriously ill prisoner and staff.

It is quite possible that these would echo the concerns of the UK prisoners, but further research in this area is needed to enable generalizations to be made. However, if we consider the causes of fear in people with life-threatening conditions, outlined by Parkes (1998a), we can see close similarities.

Fear of

- separation from loved ones, homes etc
- becoming a burden to others
- losing control
- pain, or other worsening symptoms
- being unable to complete life tasks/responsibilities
- dying
- being dead
- others (reflected fear)

Within the prison environment, it is possible that these fears would be heightened or exacerbated due to feelings of loss of control and personal autonomy experienced by many prisoners.

How then should the individual with a life-threatening condition be supported within the prison environment, and what coping mechanisms will the individual be likely to exhibit? Maull (1991) based upon the work of Kubler-Ross (1969) indicates that the following behaviours are likely to be observed:

- *Denial*—the individual focuses on early release date. If I could get out of prison, then I could have surgery and/or further treatment;
- *Anger*—there may be displacement and/or hostility shown to other prisoners and staff. If this behaviour is misinterpreted by others, then it may lead to some form of punishment;
- *Bargaining and hope*—the individual may decide to pursue litigation, become religious, or focus on release from prison with hopes of being able to pursue a course of treatment that may lead to a recovery;
- *Depression*—this is likely to have a premature onset, and may accelerate the dying process;
- *Acceptance and realization?*

How can the individual be assisted to grieve appropriately? Worden (1991) presents a four-stage model to facilitate adjustment and adaptation in bereavement:

Task 1 To accept the reality of the loss.

Task 2 To experience the pain of grief.

Task 3 To adjust to an environment without the deceased.

Task 4 To emotionally relocate the deceased and move on with life.

It is possible to adapt Worden's model to illustrate how the individual and family can be helped to adjust to a life-threatening condition within prison, as follows:

Task 1 – To accept the reality of loss

In this task we can interpret this *'reality'* as being the individual's loss of liberty and exclusion from society. This is something that may never have been properly addressed. The individual may have 'unfinished business' in relation to this, or it will, quite possibly, bring fresh feelings of resentment, anger, and frustration. Part of this frustration and anger will be borne out of the realization that they will not achieve, or complete, the life tasks or milestones that may have been realized upon release from prison. Unless the individual is able to express these feelings, supported by carers, they may not be able to grieve for this loss or subsequent losses as experienced in serious illness.

Task 2 – To experience the pain of grief

In this task the individual should be allowed to grieve as he/she chooses. There are many factors here that may inhibit the individual in expressing grief. The prison culture, for example, may mean that to exhibit emotional distress through tears is frowned upon by other prisoners and staff. It may be that grief will be expressed in other ways, such as withdrawal, attempts to self-harm, anger, hostility and displaying aggressive and abusive behaviour. The handling of such situations will need to be undertaken with sensitivity, and staff will need to be aware that this may be an expression of grief and pain, rather than disruptive behaviour liable for punishment.

Task 3 - To adjust to an environment without 'health'

As previously stated, the individual in prison has to cope with multiple losses, and now their health will have been lost as a consequence of serious illness. Parkes (1998*b*) outlines the losses associated with life-threatening illness:

- ◆ Loss of security
- ◆ Loss of physical functions
- ◆ Loss of body image
- ◆ Loss of power or strength
- ◆ Loss of self esteem

- Loss of the respect of other
- Loss of future

Parkes states that if individuals are encouraged and facilitated to express their grief at the losses that have occurred at an early stage of illness, it is more likely that they will be able to cope more effectively when they are faced with another new set of losses. It is suggested that if individuals have been facilitated to express and work through the grief caused by incarceration (as outlined above in '*Task 1*'), they should be better placed to be able to work through the losses now imposed upon them by a life-threatening illness. Coping mechanisms that may have helped them to adjust to a life inside, may now be useful to assist the individual in adjusting to life-threatening illness, and should therefore be explored.

Task 4 – To emotionally relocate the illness (and its associated losses) and move on with life

This task would reflect the impact that living with a life-threatening condition can have. We know that serious illness changes people. In some cases they describe the change for the better, in others it will have a more detrimental effect. The change that is often brought about by illness can have profound affects upon relationships with family and friends, as well as those in authority, such as prison staff. Family ties may become weaker. This may be due to the fact that family cannot cope with events as they unfold, or because the individual chooses to withdraw from family and friends. The individual may feel lost and lacking in control over circumstances, as will others previously close to the individual.

In considering this task, it is useful to draw upon the work of Stroebe (1998), who challenges Worden's linear model. Stroebe asserts that adaptation involves a process of oscillation, which involves both loss and restoration-orientated coping. Loss orientation concerns the impact of loss upon the individual, including the pain of separation, yearning, and crying about the deceased. Restoration refers to the process of adjustment that will need to take place, such as attending to life changing events, which may involve the process of learning skills that were previously undertaken by the deceased, for example, handling finances.

Within the prison context this oscillation will involve adjustment to the illness and its associated losses, such as loss of mobility. Restoration may involve denial, or avoidance of the illness in the hope of obtaining an early release date, or the development of new roles or identities as a way of adapting to life changes. Faced with, what may be for some, the reality of having to end one's life behind bars is likely to have profound effects upon relationships with carers and other prisoners. Restoration implies some sort of positive growth for the individual, and it may mean that the prisoner reviews their crime and experiences remorse, perhaps for the first time. However, it is also possible that this restoration may be negative, and bring with it hostility and anger.

Sensitive understanding from prison staff is needed to resolve the difficulties that may occur, and/or facilitation should be provided for the individual to form new roles/relationships either within existing support networks, or new networks. The message that is likely to be given out by the prisoner is '**know, respect and understand me as I am now, as an individual with health needs and concerns, rather than just another prisoner**'. What this task ultimately calls for is understanding and respect from prison staff. The individual should be allowed the opportunity to express fears and concerns without prejudice; as well as receiving the care and support that would be given to any other member of the wider population who is trying to cope with a serious illness.

Developing palliative care services for prisoners

Since the publication of the report *Patient or Prisoner* (1996) that first recommended the transfer of prison health services to the National Health Service, much has been achieved. The transfer of funding for prison health in April 2003 to the Department of Health has created a positive climate in which change can be taken forward. Prison health priorities in the United Kingdom for the period 2003–2006 include the improvement and development of primary care services, new information systems, improvements in healthcare facilities, development of the workforce as well as the strengthening of partnership working and joint planning at all levels between Primary Care Trusts, National Health Service, and prison health (Boyington 2003).

As palliative care continues to develop and extend its boundaries, the palliative needs of prisoners, who are also part of our community, should also be acknowledged and represented by health and social care providers and teams. Although no formal strategy for taking palliative care forward in prisons has been developed, there are examples of good practice appearing in recent years across the Prison Estate. Oliver and Cook (1998) described the care of a 63-year-old man admitted to the Wisdom Hospice on licence from the local prison. Whilst at the hospice his health continued to deteriorate, and he subsequently died there, but with his family present. Wilford and Holland (2002) initiated schemes to educate prison nurses in several prisons within the Trent area in pain and symptom management. HMP Kingston, recently opened the first dedicated elderly prisoner wing.

This wing is equipped to deal with the problems older prisoners present, such as mobility difficulties.

The following hypothetical case study seeks to briefly illustrate what can be done to support the prisoner, with a serious illness, who cannot be released from prison:

Case Study

Gillian is a 58-year-old prisoner. She was diagnosed with breast cancer a year ago. Unfortunately, she kept her breast lump hidden for two years. The lump was only discovered when she collapsed one day during visiting. By the time she was referred to an oncologist, her disease was too far advanced for any active treatment. She is approaching the end of her life and has recently been located on the prison hospital wing for symptom relief. She believes that her cancer is some form of punishment for her crime. She also fears for the future and that she will die alone within the prison. Gillian is serving a life sentence. The nature of her offence is such that she cannot be released, and this means that ultimately she will die in custody.

The prison approached the local palliative care provider and it was agreed that the community palliative nurses would visit the prison on a regular basis to advise on symptom management and control. The healthcare staff at the prison were supported by the community nurses to care for Gillian and additional family visits were also allowed by the Governor. Gillian eventually died one month later with a healthcare officer and close family member present.

In order to develop palliative care services for prisoners, consideration should be given to the following:

◆ Completion of a comprehensive health needs assessment of the palliative care needs of individuals within the United Kingdom prison system in order to determine the scope and need for service provision

◆ An analysis of the training and development needs of prison healthcare staff in relation to the knowledge and skills required caring for an individual with a chronic illness in prison, particularly in relation to pain and symptom management, encompassing the palliative care approach

◆ Development of an appropriate skill mix that will facilitate the development of a palliative care team structure, supported by appropriate networks and partnerships with primary care teams and voluntary agencies and others

◆ Adaptation and implementation of standard protocols of care, particularly in relation to the availability and utilization of controlled drugs. Consideration should also be given to the development of integrated care pathways to facilitate equity and consistency in health care services

◆ Planned programmes of research that focus on the evaluation of the patient/prisoner experience of receiving palliative care services in order to steer the way forward for the development of programmes of care in this unique and challenging environment.

Conclusion

Death and dying within prison will present significant challenges for the individual with a life-threatening condition, families, loved ones, prison staff as well as other prisoners. A prison sentence will result in a number of significant losses for the individual and family. Such losses are likely to be exacerbated by periods of illness, and there will be new and even greater losses that will have to be endured if the illness becomes life threatening. In attempting to adapt and cope with such losses the individual may exhibit a number of different coping strategies and mechanisms. Individuals in prison, with a chronic illness, can be helped to adjust to their changing circumstances and condition if supported by carers to share their fears and concerns.

A positive movement for change has now been created following the transfer of funds for prison health to the Department of Health. Palliative care providers and National Health Services should form positive partnerships to consider how best the needs of the palliative prisoner can be met to ensure that the individual who is socially excluded is still afforded the basic human right to a death with dignity and minimal suffering, similar to any other member of the wider community.

References

Boyington J (2003) Prison Health—The Future Vision. *Prison Health Newsletter. Department of Health* 12:1–3.

British Medical Association (2001) *Prison Medicine: A Crisis Waiting to Break.* BMA, London.

British Medical Association Medical Ethics Committee (1996) *Guidance for Doctors Providing Medical Care and Treatment to those Detained in Prison.* BMA, London.

British Medical Association (1993) *Medical Ethics Today: Its Practice and Philosophy.* BMJ Publishing Group United Kingdom, Great Britain.

Coyle A (2001) The purposes of imprisonment. In Bryans S and Jones R (ed.) *Prisons and the Prisoner: An Introduction to the Work of Her Majesty's Prison Service.* HMSO, Norwich.

Department of Health (1999) *The Future Organisation of Prison Health Care.* Report by the Joint Prison Service and National Health Service Executive Working Group. DOH, London.

Faull C (1998) The history and principles of palliative care. In Faull C, Carter Y, and Woof R (ed.) *Handbook of Palliative Care*. Blackwell Science Ltd, London.

Fursland E (1999) 'Inside Job' *Nursing Times* **95**(37):24–6.

Her Majesty's Chief Inspector of Prisons (1999) *Report of an Unannounced Inspection of Wormwood Scrubs: 8–12 March* Home Office, London.

Her Majesty's Chief Inspector of Prisons (1996) *Patient or Prisoner. A New Strategy for Health Care in Prisons.* Home Office, London.

Lemieux CM, Dyeson TB, and Castiglione B (2002) Revisiting the Literature on Prisoners Who are Older: Are We Wiser? *The Prison Journal* **82**(4):440–58.

Matthews R (1999) *Doing Time: An Introduction to the Sociology of Imprisonment.* Palgrave, Basingstoke.

Maull F (1991) Dying in prison: sociocultural and psychosocial dynamics. *The Hospice Journal* **7**:1/2 127–41.

McManus J (2001) *Better Health, Lower Crime: A Briefing for the NHS and Partner Agencies.* National Association for the Care and Resettlement of Offenders, London.

Newell M (2003) A New Paradigm of Decarceration. *Prison Service Journal* **150**:2–8.

Oliver D and Cook L (1998) The Specialist Palliative Care of Prisoners. *European Journal of Palliative Care* **5**(3):79–80.

Parkes CM (1998*a*) Coping with loss: facing loss. *British Medical Journal* **316**:1521–4.

Parkes CM (1998*b*) Coping with loss: the dying adult. *British Medical Journal* **316**:1313–15.

Ratcliff M (2002) Hospice care for prisoners—the US experience. *Hospice Information Bulletin* **1**(3):1–2.

Ratcliff M (2000) Dying inside the walls. *Innovations in End-of-Life Care* **2**(3), www.edc.org/lastacts (accessed 13/01/03).

Reed J and Lyne M (1997) The quality of health care in prison: results of a year's programme of semi-structured inspections. *British Medical Journal* **315**:1420–4.

Smith R (1997) Prisoners: an end to second class health care? *British Medical Journal* **318**:954–5.

Stroebe M (1998) New directions in bereavement research: exploration of gender differences. *Palliative Medicine* **12**:5–12.

Tillman T (2000) The psychological needs of the terminally ill patient in a prison environment. *Innovations in End-of-Life Care* **2**(3) www.edc.org/lastacts (accessed 13/01/03).

United Kingdom Central Council for Nursing, Midwifery and Health Visiting (1999) *Nursing in Secure Environments.* United Kingdom, London.

Worden W (1991) *Grief Counselling and Grief Therapy. (2nd Ed)* Routledge, London.

Wilford T and Holland L (2002) Palliative care in prisons. *Macmillan Information Exchange,* (September) 6.

World Health Organisation (1998) *Health in Prisons Project.* Consensus Statement On Mental Health Promotion in Prisons. The Hague. WHO.

10

Refugees

Mary Blanche and Chris Endersby

Introduction

Writing a contribution focused upon refugees and palliative care services is in many ways very timely. There is a wealth of literature around both subjects, yet there is only a limited range of resources that provide connections between the two areas. Despite much of the recent media and political attention in Western Europe, the movement of refugees is not a new phenomenon. Much of the information included within this chapter relates to issues that have affected individuals' access to and experience of health and social care services over a considerable length of time. It is also likely that the challenges and opportunities related to providing responsive services within this context will continue to be of relevance in the long-term. This chapter is written to promote discussion and raise awareness for practitioners and those working in areas allied to palliative care services, of some of the issues related to refugees.

There is an increasing amount of information and plenty of myths in the public arena related to refugees and asylum seekers. This chapter makes use of several case examples to identify issues that are relevant to understanding 'refugee experiences' and palliative care services. The relationship between health, behaviour, and experience is complex and identifying the impact of the 'refugee experience' upon health, within personal biographies that may also include factors related to minority status, ethnicity, culture, religion, language, and gender, is a difficult task. The chapter commences by offering an insight into the terms associated with refugees.

Refugees—definitions and diversities

Refugees have been formally identified and recognized as an identifiable group within the world's migrant population since the passing of the UN

Convention in 1951 and its associated 1967 protocol. As such, definitions of and responses to refugees emerged at a similar time to the hospice movement and literature related to palliative care (Hockley 1999). The convention produced a relatively narrow definition of 'refugee' and placed the burden of evidence upon individuals to demonstrate a 'well-founded fear of persecution'.

> A refugee is a person who 'owing to a well-founded fear of being persecuted for reasons of race, religion, nationality, membership of a particular social group, or political opinion, is outside the country of his nationality, and is unable to or, owing to such fear, is unwilling to avail himself of the protection of that country...'
>
> The 1951 Convention relating to the Status of Refugees (UNHCR 1996)

The UN Convention was not intended to respond to the movement of people following natural disasters (earthquakes, floods, or famine). Even some forms of social catastrophes that may result within a region following civil unrest or conflict may not guarantee recognition of refugee status. However since this time, the role of the United Nations High Commission for Refugees (UNHCR) that was established through these provisions has seen its work expand into such areas. There are 144 individual states that have ratified the Convention; however, there are wide ranging interpretations of their duties and responsibilities under the 1951 Convention (UNHCR 2000 and 2002). The convention does not afford protection to internally displaced persons and does not guarantee that claims for asylum will be recognized by governments, as rights for refugees commence on acceptance of a relevant claim. The principle expression of these rights is that of non-refoulement (not forcibly returning individuals to countries where they may face persecution).

In January 2002, the UNHCR identified in excess of 19.8 million migrants (including potential and former refugees) about whom they had concern. The UNHCR indicates that in 2002 there were approximately 12 million refugees, with 384,530 individuals claiming asylum in the European Union (EU) during 2001. Individuals who have their refugee status formally acknowledged by a government in the industrialized world are a small minority of the world's migrant population, the vast majority of whom find 'refuge' much closer to home. Many refugees desire an eventual return to home. For these refugees a diagnosis of terminal illness may mean giving up the dream of returning home or returning home quickly possibly to inadequate health service.

In addition to people who have had their refugee status formally recognized by government, this chapter includes within its understanding of 'refugee', those individuals awaiting decisions (asylum seekers) and people still residing in the host country while engaging with appeals processes. Also included are those individuals who are granted leave to remain, or temporary admission in its variety of forms. Illnesses that may result in the need to access palliative care services may be relevant to alternative 'humanitarian' provisions available to a government, however only in very specific experiences would it relate to the merit of their claim for refugee status.

Responses to refugees at a European and domestic level

The area of immigration was at the heart of ideals around European co-operation in the post-war era that saw the passing of the European Convention on Human Rights. Alongside such ideals there has also have been wide ranging concerns expressed about immigration. These have ranged from sovereignty to concerns about the very social, economic, and political fabric of society and how this has been affected by widespread migration. While great strides were made to improve the freedom of trade, movement of people across the union and the creation of universal rights for citizens of Europe, the desire to control entry to the community has been equally strong (Levy 1999 pp. 12–13). As many of the internal borders have come down, allowing freedom of movement across the EU, so compensatory forces have seen the external controls increased, leading many authors and commentators to use the phrase 'Fortress Europe' (Harding 2000; Dummett 2001). At the same time that the EU is expanding, it will be working to secure common responses to refugees and asylum seekers as the perceived 'burden' of such populations are shared across the Union's members. A concern is that states will seek to agree upon the lowest common denominator in terms of provision of support and acceptance of claims—the so-called 'rush for the bottom' (Lavenex 2001). This may deny refugees the opportunity to make claims, or benefit from necessary humanitarian assistance when they enter states.

Despite issues related to asylum and refugees coming to the fore in the past few years in the UK, the country has provided a refuge for people fleeing their own countries for centuries. The movement of people into the UK has been a characteristic of the 20th century. The First World War, the Spanish civil war, and the Second World War all saw arrivals of refugees. The second half of the century has also seen significant movements of persons into the UK from Communist States, Uganda, Chile, Vietnam, Kosova, Rwanda, Sri Lanka, Afghanistan, Kurdish regions, and Zimbabwe. This list is far from exhaustive and does not indicate the heterogeneous characteristic of each of these populations themselves, with refugees often originating from minority populations within each society. There have been marked differences in the demographics of these populations, but the personal biographies of many older refugees may lead to difficulties in adjusting to new relationships, which may be highlighted in the terminal phase of an illness. Refugees may find it hard to accept the help of palliative care staff.

The British Government has sought to control passage across its borders since passing the 1905 Aliens Act. Through successive legislation, the principle of providing refuge has been maintained within the context of controlling inward migration, through the imposition of visa requirements, financial penalties to carriers, and internal disincentives such as detention and restriction to benefit. Fernando (2002) highlights that due to these measures most migrants in the later part of the 20th century are asylum seekers and refugees and that their arrival has rarely been met with a favourable attitude (Fernando 2002). Even prior to the recent, increasingly restrictive nature of immigration legislation, as applied to potential refugees, Solomos identified the disproportionate impact of such provisions upon the basis of religion, race, ethnicity and colour (Solomos 1989).

In recent years, it would have been difficult to miss the 'social' understandings afforded to refugees and asylum seekers. At the time of writing this chapter, the public discourse extends from concerns around the personal safety of individuals through potential communication of infectious diseases, such as SARS, to the risk from potential terrorists within the population.

These not only impact upon the operation of individual prejudice but also add further weight to moves to exclude potential asylum seekers and refugees (even prior to arrival in the UK through establishing reception facilities outside of the EU where claims can be assessed prior to entry).

Refugees, health, and health services

In a recent report authored by the British Medical Association into meeting the healthcare needs of asylum seekers, the lack of research related to the health problems of asylum seekers at arrival was highlighted. Also explored was the potentially limited effectiveness of screening at arrival. Additionally, the report indicated that little is known about health difficulties emerging after significant time in the UK (BMA 2002).

Refugee children may have been born during flight, at the time of arrival in the host country, or may have arrived unaccompanied (those children and young people claiming asylum without the care and protection of their parents account for approximately 5% of the total population). Refugees who have reason to make use of palliative care services may have been resident in the country for some time, while others may have known of this need prior to their flight, during the course of their journey or at the time of arrival.

For others their move may have been made in later stages of life. The timing of such moves may be significant to individuals, and this contributes to the range of life experiences that demand services to be responsive to individuals rather than based upon assumptions. Nazroo (1997) explores the difficulty of definition of immigrants when studying the health of ethnic minorities, identifying the impact of the migration experience upon indicators of health and illness in both the host country and that of origin as a complex issue (Nazroo 1997).

Marks and Hilder (1997) in their comparative study of Jewish and Bengali immigrants in and around Spitlefields, East London identified the assumption that migrants' health will be poorer than that of the indigenous population. They identified higher mortality rates in country of origin and the difficulty in accessing health and social care services as reasons for this, while viewing demographic and economic mobility as potentially producing moderating influences (Marks and Hilder 1997). Religion and culture may further impact upon health related behaviours, such as abstention from drink or smoking. Therefore, just as it is important to treat each patient as an individual, so it is important to treat refugees as individual people with their needs distinct and often separate from their asylum status.

The complex nature of competing hypotheses of 'selection' and 'stress' that are identified and explored by Littlewood *et al.* (1999) and Nazroo (1997) present further considerations for professionals and services responding to the health needs of refugees. The selection hypothesis asserts that individuals fleeing the country of origin are different on the basis of demography and socio-economic factors, leading to the more influential or affluent individuals leaving. It is also possible however that those in societies with the greatest mobility are those who may be the most isolated and their flight may well be the result of economic and social pressures that have been operating for some time. The stress hypothesis indicates that the process of migration is in itself stressful and that many difficulties faced by refugees are related to their movement and thereby direct comparisons with the population in the host country or that of origin may not be straightforward. The movement of persons, their motivations, ability to control their flight, passage, and circumstances related to their arrival are extremely diverse and therefore the implication of these experiences upon health are complex and again require practitioners to adopt a wide perspective when interpreting health related behaviour.

The WHO Europe report, exploring a range of social determinants of health asserts that a wide range of social factors strongly affect health throughout life. The messages of the report can all be related to experiences facing refugees, who are often socially excluded and face many challenges that may be cumulative in their effect (Wilkinson and Marmot 1998).

In discussing palliative care in India, Burn (1997) highlights the following barriers to accessing care services: poverty, fear, ignorance of the disease process, lack of information regarding treatment options, communication difficulties, and long distances to travel to and from the hospital. Firth (1993) identified that recently arrived immigrants' unfamiliarity with the medical, social and legal system, lack of understanding of procedures, communication difficulties, and difference in religious and social support from their own communities, contribute to difficulties around access (Firth 1993). The chapter progresses by exploring the broad categories as highlighted by Burn (1997) and applying these to refugees in the UK.

Poverty (socio-economic factors)

Part of the public discourse around asylum seekers is their intention to seek economic advantage through arrival in the industrialized world. The reality of support afforded to asylum seekers places them below basic levels of subsistence in many European countries. Asylum seekers are excluded from accessing many supplemental forms of support (e.g. social fund loans, disability living allowance, and funeral grants). This is compounded by difficulty in ensuring access to support to which they are entitled (Penrose 2002). The presumption in offering this lower level of support, as Penrose highlights, was that asylum seekers would only be subject to such processes on a short-term basis. This has not taken account of the wide variation in the length of time for a decision to be reached for individuals (Penrose 2002). Support via vouchers was further criticized for reducing ability of families to shop around for produce and having a social stigma that saw such families set apart from others in need of assistance.

Recent changes in the UK, introduced by the 2002 Nationality, Immigration & Asylum Act, will potentially deny asylum seekers any form of financial assistance or accommodation support and also prevents asylum seekers from working while awaiting a decision on their claim. Asylum seekers will therefore be increasingly dependent upon support and assistance that is self-accessed through informal networks of community support. For those asylum seekers refusing dispersal (a single offer of accommodation is offered) no financial support is made available.

The present system that prevents asylum seekers from working may impose additional dependency upon services and support. Gaining status as a 'refugee' does not guarantee entitlements, or the means to make the transition to independence, as those statutory agencies funded to support asylum seekers are unable to claim for work with refugees.

Fear

Many asylum seekers and refugees fear contact with people in authority. This is a realistic fear when we consider that the principle basis of a claim for refugee status to be recognized is related to actions of authority figures and institutions. Refugees are likely to have been viewed as at odds with authority in their country of origin. Some of them have first hand experience of torture at the hands of the authorities and in certain regimes the medical profession and institutions, however unwilling, may have played a part in the torture that refugees experienced. In another culture, speaking a different language and with a very varied experience of healthcare and potentially different conception of illness, asylum seekers and refugees may avoid hospital care and may view hospice workers as authority. For those individuals living 'illegally' within the host country, contact with hospitals may mean detection and therefore deportation, which may mean a refusal to access medical care, even in times of emergency. The authors have first hand experience of a boy with a serious injury who did not seek treatment because the hospitals as state agencies were run by perceived enemies.

It will not be unusual for refugees to tell palliative care staff very little about their background and history or for alternative narratives to be offered. Trust can come with time and individuals may divulge more information as they gain more knowledge of the respect for confidentiality. Professionals must accept the possibility of encountering several different narratives that may possibly conflict. The verification of information, the potential to obtain important medical data related to previous treatment may also be hard to obtain, however the authors have known clients arrive with medical notes related to previously diagnosed conditions.

Refugees may already have experienced considerable trauma and loss associated with their experiences prior to or during flight, which may lead to previous events dominating their daily lives. This can make acceptance of and planning for their own future care challenging. This may potentially continue for a significant time after the legal processes around their claim have been concluded.

Individual asylum seekers may also have fears about the success of their asylum claim. Refugees may view their illness either as a vulnerability which may save them from deportation or as a factor which will make deportation more likely. Perceptions of powerlessness and hopelessness associated with the resolution of claims and the limits to self-determination may well be debilitating when facing fears around illness. Working together to establish and resolve practical issues unrelated to either their status as a refugee (or indeed to their presenting medical needs) may be a solid basis for a later, more focused relationship. Assistance with such tasks may enable a constructive relationship to develop, which values the importance of the refugee's existing coping-strategies. This is likely to evoke a sense of 'partnership' which may well be essential in the construction of shared knowledge about beliefs, experiences, and perceptions of health, illness and decision making.

The impact of fear on the part of the caregiver cannot be ignored as a potential barrier to competent care. At a time when media headlines often equate asylum seekers with health concerns, crime, or terrorism, professional caregivers may need to acknowledge and address their feelings and attitudes towards patients who also wear the label 'asylum seeker'. Much has been written about 'prejudice' and 'discrimination' within both medical and social care literature. The impact of large family groups within institutions or the wish to access alternative, culturally specific 'healing processes', may all challenge services and professionals. Accepting that such issues exist within services and between professionals, service users and their clients, will enable creative solutions to be promoted that meet the needs of all concerned (Firth 1993).

The following case study illustrates not just the problems facing refugees in accessing palliative care services, but also the psychological difficulties that can be encountered in dealing with the illness without the support of friends and family.

Case Study

'Clothilde was born in the Democratic Republic of the Congo. She was the older of two sisters and she lived with her family in a small village. When Clothilde was small, her parents owned some land in the village and they were considered to be relatively prosperous. However, hostile factions within the village took advantage of the general disintegration of Congolese society to take parcels of land and raise crops on them. There was very little that Clothilde's parents could do to prevent this but Clothilde's father did protest to the village council. The protest was unsuccessful and resulted in bad feeling between Clothilde's family and other villagers.

One day, when Clothilde was 16 years old, she was coming back from the fields and some of the young men from the village attacked her. Clothilde was raped. This is often done to give a warning to families. Clothilde's parents were very upset when they realised that she had been attacked although she never revealed the exact nature of the assault to them. Her parents decided that all three daughters must leave and they paid a large sum of money to friends to help them.

On the journey to the UK, Clothilde became separated from one of her sisters and arrived in the UK with her younger sister aged 12. By the time they reached the UK, Clothilde was feeling unwell. Both she and her sister were placed in the care of the local authority. Clothilde was sad and unwell. She missed her parents and felt that she had let them down by becoming separated from her younger sister. Her foster parents were kind but their food was unfamiliar and unappetising and only their youngest son, aged 20, spoke competent French. Sometimes the Social Worker arranged for a French interpreter but it was often a different interpreter on each occasion.

After months in the UK, Clothilde had become a diligent student with a reasonable understanding of English. She remained unwell and an unexplained weight loss promoted her foster mother to take her to the doctor. At this point, she was diagnosed as HIV positive. Feeling isolated and not wishing to upset her remaining younger sister, Clothilde presents as depressed and incommunicative and does not comply with her drugs regime. She has refused to contact her parents, as she is ashamed of her situation. Her asylum status remains unresolved.'

In seeking to help Clothilde, we would need to be aware of her feelings of shame and embarrassment. Contact with the Refugee Council advisors may help to lessen her isolation and increase our knowledge of her cultural needs.

Ignorance of the 'disease' process

Asylum seekers and refugees may be perceived to be ignorant of the disease process in western terms that emphasize the predominance of medical and scientific knowledge, but may merely be defining the disease process in the light of their own cultural understanding and experience.

> Culture has been described as a 'set of guidelines (both explicit and implicit) which individuals inherit as members of a particular society and which tells them how to view the world, how to experience it emotionally and how to behave in relation to other people, to supernatural forces or gods and to the natural environment'
>
> (Helman 2000).

Donald (1998) indicates that the 'western' narrative of disease in terms of the identification, causation, and treatment and the power of the medical profession can conflict with the personal experience and expression of illness (Donald 1998). Allen (1996) suggests that the Mali people of Uganda saw the Aids virus, which accelerated at the time of the civil war, as a 'poison' which was encompassed by beliefs drawn from witchcraft, Christianity, and biomedicine. Barlow (1992) reports that many ethnic minority women are affected by religious or social barriers in seeking treatment for Aids and she reports that women from sub-Saharan Africa often present late for services.

Many refugees may have had years without effective health care. Their journeys to countries of safety may have been long and arduous punctuated by periods where they may have spent time working in order to gain resources for the next leg of their journey. In these circumstances, healthcare is often unobtainable and the refugee's general health is likely to be neglected. A recent health assessment pilot in East Kent (Ann Farebrother, personal correspondence to author) found little evidence of major health problems in asylum seekers arriving in the UK. However, general poor health in relation to dental care, skin problems, and evidence of malnutrition is relatively common. As the BMA report indicates however, little is known about later presentation of health difficulties and as time progresses and claims are resolved, it is likely that specific projects and workers originally involved will withdraw due to funding restrictions and competing demands upon their services (BMA 2002).

Lack of information regarding treatment options

Refugees are particularly susceptible to gaps in information regarding a whole range of necessary services. Many previous studies have also highlighted the marginalized status of black and minority health provision within the National Health Service. The recent Sainsbury Centre report 'Breaking the Circles of Fear' called for a comprehensive review and analysis related to the experiences of mental health services by people from ethnic minorities (SCMH 2002). This group of palliative care services users are likely to be doubly disadvantaged, by not having a clear understanding of health service processes. Roberts (2000) argues that 'asylum seekers and refugees with a disability remain invisible because of a failure to recognise that some asylum seekers whose identities encompass ... those of refugees, disabled people and minority ethnic groups remain lost because they are not recognized by either the refugee community (because of their impairment) or by the disability movement (because of the immigration status)' (Roberts 2000).

There are significant health issues related to the routine detention of asylum seekers. In the UK, increasing numbers of asylum seekers, including children living within families, are detained. Detention adds to psychosocial stressors, potentially resulting in anxiety, depression, and other psychiatric illness (Pourgourides *et al.* 1996 and HM Inspector of Prisons 2003).

Communication will also be an issue, as many asylum seekers will have a limited knowledge of English as a second language. Hill and Penso (1995) identified a lack of translated materials in relevant languages in both hospital and hospice services and a dearth of interpreting services. These problems are likely to be even more prevalent in relation to asylum seekers who are unlikely to originate from an ethnic group already settled in the area and for whom such material may well be prepared. This is likely to be so in part because of the dispersal process. Burnett and Fassil (2000) provide a comprehensive digest of practical considerations related to culture and communication for health professionals.

Watters (2000) identified that refugee women may face additional isolation, with potentially less education than men and fewer opportunities to learn English. Additionally women may arrive in the host country without their partners and this may place them in fear and isolation from both the host community as well as their refugee community.

As Firth (2001) notes, care should be taken to use adequate and appropriate interpreting services rather than other family members. However, the interpreter's own attitude to and experience of illness and dying may need to be explored in order to ensure that the interpreter is comfortable with the material being discussed. It is also important that staff working through interpreters are clear about the appropriate pace and diction of their speech. Equally, when using an interpreter there may be occasions where the use of a particular gender for interpreting is preferred for cultural and personal reasons.

Long distance from hospital

This may become a particular issue for asylum seekers in the UK following the Nationality, Immigration & Asylum Act 2002 and the establishment of large accommodation centres for people awaiting decisions on asylum status. The Government will provide medical support within the centres but there will not be hospital facilities. Combined with the increasing tendency towards specialist cancer care centres, this may mean that asylum seekers have to travel long distances for appropriate treatments.

Case Study

Georg left Hungary at the time of the Hungarian uprising in 1956. He was 20 years old and a student at Budapest University and took to the streets when the Russian tanks came over the borders. Defeated, he left Hungary and made his way to the UK where he successfully claimed asylum.

He was unable to contact his parents for many years and when he did so, it was to discover that his father had died in the intervening years. His mother remained in Hungary but Georg's siblings were scattered throughout the world. Georg managed to establish a life in England and he married an English woman when he was in his early thirties. He failed, however, to complete his studies and he worked as a security guard in a factory until his retirement at the age of 65. Georg and his wife, Judy, had two children, Sally and Paul but Georg was a remote father. He never forgot his early hardships and worked long hours to give the family a secure life style. He was often over critical of his children, contrasting their life with the life he had to lead as a child and young adult. Judy died suddenly three years ago and Georg became more and more isolated from his adult children.

Recently, Georg was diagnosed as suffering from lung cancer having smoked throughout his life. He presents as quite isolated, his relationship with his children is quite formal and he has no other close friends. His relationships with former work colleagues faded long ago.

Georg does not talk much but he has begun increasingly to mention his life as a child in Hungary to his palliative care nurse. He appears to be wistful on such occasions.

Refugees who have apparently successfully integrated may find illness exacerbates earlier feeling of isolation. It may be helpful to explore past memories of their original country. A few suitable words or phrases from their first language may show courtesy and concern. This is often available on the internet.

Conclusions

The case studies illustrate that refugees approach palliative care services in a variety of ways. Although asylum seekers and refugees are often acknowledged in the western world as being a relatively new phenomenon, people have sought safety from both political and economic insecurity for generations. It is, therefore, as likely that palliative care staff will encounter refugees with an emotional history of loss and adaptation, as they will encounter current asylum seekers facing adjustments and community hostility.

If effective care that acknowledges the whole of the individual is to be given, it is important to remember:

◆ Refugees, like every other patient, deserve to have their cultural needs met and to be treated with respect and dignity. As always, the patient or their family are often best suited to outlining these needs. Internet searches for country of origin information may also yield useful advice for staff and enable a fuller understanding of the issues facing the individual.

◆ Staff have to face their own prejudices. Information from organizations like the Red Cross and the Refugee Council may be valuable in enabling staff to confront their own fears and see the person beyond the statistics.

◆ Care should be taken to give clear messages of welcome to all minority groups. A multi-cultural staff and volunteer group can help to lessen feelings of isolation. Some organizations may feel able to approach refugee organizations to offer volunteering opportunities to their members that may extend to staff training.

◆ Access to professional interpreters may be crucial. This will not only aid medical and nursing care but will also ensure that the patient is aware of the whole range of palliative care services available.

◆ Past feelings of loss may be reawakened in the terminal phase of any illness and many refugees will have unresolved losses. Equally, the lack of family members and shared history may make bereavement difficult (Walter 1999).

◆ Consideration should be given to the translation of appropriate documents to aid patient access.

◆ Refugees have often told their life story many times to many different people for many different reasons. It is important when working with them to try not to ask intrusive questions, accepting narratives with respect, and acknowledging that these may be later revised and revisited.

◆ Care should be taken in physical examination of refugees that cultural mores are respected, reluctance to participate in such examinations may also stem from past history of unwanted physical attention or abuse. This reluctance can be framed in different ways and should be handled sensitively. It may be necessary to undertake such examinations over time as trust is gained, with chaperones offered and issues related to gender considered.

In caring for asylum seekers and refugees, we should seek to acknowledge and celebrate their cultural diversity, to give them support which shows them that the host community values them and to help them face their illness in a way which feels appropriate and comfortable to them. For this to happen, all staff need not only to adhere to principles and values associated to working in partnership with service users and their families, but also to acknowledge the potential fundamental differences in understanding and coping with matters related to health, illness, mortality, spirituality, and metaphysical issues. These may raise questions for all involved of how to adapt palliative care services to be responsive to the 'holistic' needs of such a diverse population.

References

Allen T (1996) A flight from refuge. In Allen T (ed.) *In Search of Cool Ground: War, Flight & Homecoming in North East Africa*, pp. 220–6. James Currey, London.

BMA (2002) *Asylum Seekers: Meeting their Healthcare Needs*. BMA, London.

Barlow J (1992) Social issues: an overview. In Morrison V and McLachlan S (ed.) *Working with Women and Aids, Bury*. Tavistock Routledge, London.

Burn G (1997) Development of palliative care in India. In Saunders and Kastenbaum (ed.) *Hospice Care on the International Scene*. Springer Publishing Co, New York.

Burnett A and Fassil Y (2000) *Meeting the Health Needs of Refugees and Asylum Seekers in the UK; An Information and Resource Pack for Health Workers*. NHS, London.

Donald A (1998) The words we live in. In Greenhalgh T and Hurwitz B (ed.) *Narrative Based Medicine; Dialogue & Discourse in Clinical Practice*. BMJ, London.

Dummett M (2001) *On Immigration and Refugees*. Routledge, London.

Fernando S (2002) *Mental Health, Race and Culture*, (2nd edn). Palgrave, New York.

Firth S (1993) Cultural issues in terminal care. In Clark D (ed.) *The Future of Palliative Care; Issues of Policy & Practice*. Open University Press, Buckingham.

Firth S (2001) Wider horizons—care of the dying in a multicultural society National Council for Hospice and Specialist Palliative Care Services.

HM Inspector of Prisons (2003) *Introduction & Summary of Findings Inspection of Five Immigration Service custodial Establishments*. The Home Office, London.

Harding J (2000) *The Uninvited; Refugees at the Rich Man's Gate*. Profile Books, London.

Helman C (2000) *Culture, Health and Illness: an Introduction for Health Practitioners* (4th edn). Hodder Arnold, London.

Hill D and Penso D (1995) Opening doors—improving access to hospice and specialist palliative care services by members of the Black & Ethnic Minority Community, NCHSPCS

Hockley J (1999) The Evolution of the Hospice Approach. In Clark D, Hockley S, and Ahmedzai S (eds.) *New Themes in Palliative Care*. Open University Press, Buckingham.

Lavenex S (2001) *The Europeanisation of Refugee Policies; Between Human Rights and Internal Security*. Aldershot, Ashgate.

Levy C (1999) European asylum and refugee policy after the Treaty of Amsterdam: the birth of a new regime? In Bloch A and Levy C (ed.) *Refugees, Citizenship and Social Policy in Europe*. Palgrave, Hamps.

Littlewood R and Lipsedge M (1999) *Aliens and Alienists: Ethnic Minorities and Psychiatry*. Routledge, London.

Marks L and Hilder L (1997) Ethnic advantage; infant survival among Jewish & Bengali immigrants in East London 1870–1990. In Marks L and Worboys M (ed.) *Migrants, Minorities and Health; Historical & Contemporary Studies*. Routledge, London.

Nazroo J (1997) *Ethnicity and Mental Health: Findings from a National Community Survey*. Policy Studies Institute, London.

Penrose J (2002) *Poverty and Asylum in the UK*. Oxfam & The Refugee Council, London.

Pourgourides C, Sashidharan S and Bracken P (1996) *A Second Exile; The Mental Health Implications of Detention of Asylum Seekers in the United Kingdom, Northern Birmingham Mental Health NHS Trust*. University of Birmingham & The Barrow Cadbury Trust.

Roberts K (2000) Lost in the system? *Disabled Refugees and Asylum Seekers in Britain in Disability & Society* **15**(6): 943–48.

Sainsbury Centre for Mental Health (2002) *Breaking the Circles of Fear; A Review of the Relationship Between Mental Health Services and the African & Caribbean Communities*. SCMH, London.

Solomos J (1989) *Race and Racism in Contemporary Britain*. Macmillan, Hamps.

UNHCR (1996) *Convention and Protocol Related to the Status of Refugees*. United Nations High Commission for Refugees, Geneva.

UNHCR (2000) *The State of the World's Refugees 2000—Fifty Years of Humanitarian Action*. Oxford University Press, Oxford.

UNHCR (2002) Refugees by numbers 2002, UNHCR (*www.unchr.ch* accessed April 2003).

Walter T (1999) *The Mourning for Diana*. Berg. Publishers Ltd.

Watters C (2000) The need for understanding, Health Matters, No. 39 Winter 1999/2000 (*www.healthmatters.org.uk/stories/watters.html* accessed April 2003)

Wilkinson R and Marmot M (1998) *Social Determinants of Health; The Solid Facts*. WHO Europe.

11

Finances

Donal Gallagher

Those affected by serious illness and bereavement encounter a range of changes and losses. How personal finances feature in these experiences has received scant attention within the literature (Gallagher 2002). Money is key in the healthy population's measurement of quality of life (Ferriss 2002) and in spite of the potential for changed perspectives there is every chance that those facing death or bereavement will continue to see finances as a determinant of their well being. Whilst the availability of money in itself represents a tangible example of socio-economic status, it is often linked in studies to other social profiling factors such as employment, housing, and education. Together these have been used to identify an individual's poverty level (Blane *et al.* 1998). Furthermore, a person's health and relationship with the health care system is greatly dictated by their socio-economic status. This structural perspective will be examined before focusing on the ramifications of changed personal finances on the lives of the seriously ill and the bereaved. Subsequently the implications for services and practitioners working with these clients* will be discussed. In doing so it is recognized that much work is carried out with this client group by professionals and volunteers in non-specialist palliative care services including community health teams, respiratory teams, and voluntary bereavement services. The emphasis within the chapter will be on specialist palliative care teams due to the bias in the literature and the author's practice experience but it is intended that the points raised will be more widely relevant.

Income, health, and bereavement

More is understood about the effect of social class on health than any other variable (Blane *et al.* 1998). Essentially those living in poverty are more

---

*The term client will be used throughout this chapter for ease of reference to those with a terminal illness, those close to them and the bereaved.

likely to become ill and develop certain types of illnesses. In behavioural terms the greater incidence of smoking among the lower social classes predisposes them to developing lung cancer. This unmistakable and well-known relationship is recognized by those designing social and health care policies as they strive to ensure that a lack of social improvements or effective targeting of services does not undermine the benefits of advances in treatment and medical technology. In the United Kingdom, one of the aims of the NHS Cancer Plan is to 'tackle the inequalities in health that mean unskilled workers are twice as likely to die from cancer as professionals' (NHS 2000). 'Joined up thinking' is being employed in government initiatives to reduce poverty levels which are not only justifiable in themselves but are expected to impact on other associated forms of social exclusion: 'poorer health, homelessness, and earlier death' (Bevan 2002).

Palliative care organizations have set an agenda for reaching groups who have been unable or unwilling to access the care they provide (National Council 2001) and in so doing have looked at how the 'disadvantaged dying' (Clark and Seymour 1999) can be encompassed within their remit. In spite of the alleged non-discriminatory nature of cancer, the evidence suggests that many of the potential recipients of palliative care services will come from the poorer sections of society (Blane *et al.* 1998). This greater health need is not matched by shorter waiting times or better access to elective treatments in the NHS (Pettinger 1999) and lower income also reduces the chances of someone dying at home (Hunt 1997). The needs, values, and experiences of individuals within this group must be understood and reacted to if disadvantage is not to be compounded by unresponsive services and a lack of genuine choice.

Does the fact that someone has less financial resources pre-dispose them to a more distressing bereavement? The lack of agreement about this (Parkes 1990) has been altered subsequently by a few studies that looked at this factor, leading to an acknowledgement that a lower income can disadvantage the bereaved (Landau 1995; Wyatt *et al.* 1999). As a result this is now reflected as an element to be considered in deciding risk in bereavement (Relf 2000). From what has been presented earlier it is also evident that not only will those in poorer sections of society experience death in their family at a younger age but their life experience prior to this event is more likely to have contained socially determined forms of loss and disadvantage.

Low income can have a significant effect on whether someone develops a serious illness and their subsequent relationship with the health care system. Those surviving a death can also be excluded by their social circumstances. The changes associated with ill health and bereavement can exacerbate the situation for those living on a low income and introduce others to new social losses. Loss is linked with pain and this form of pain will now be discussed.

Financial pain

The totality of care underlying palliative care services' philosophy commits them not only to understanding the past, present, and future elements of clients' lives but also their diversity of need. The richness of the research into these needs is impoverished by the paucity of studies about the social concerns of clients. Recent writing has helped in both drawing attention to the emphasis placed on the emotional and psychological elements of psychosocial care and in focusing on social pain (Field 2000; Wright *et al.* 2002; Sheldon 2003). Nevertheless Sheldon's comment that this 'is the least-understood aspect of 'total pain'' remains true (2003). The lack of knowledge about how social factors and in particular income effect bereavement is even more striking. The results of any research that has included financial concerns are flavoured by their almost exclusive use of cancer patients as subjects and the reliance on patients from different parts of the disease trajectory (Soothill *et al.* 2001*a, b*). Moreover, the fact that many of the studies were conducted in the USA with its variable health care funding arrangements will exert a particular influence on the outcomes. Relying on the research will help us to a degree. Drawing on what clients have to say will enhance our understanding significantly.

Case Study

Gary (45) is married to Helen (43) and they have 2 children, Ben (12), who is autistic and Rebecca (10). Gary has been diagnosed with bowel cancer. He has always worked for an engineering company and rarely needed to take time off through sickness until he developed cancer. When the social worker first went to meet Gary and Helen they spent a long time talking about the recent 'devastating' news that the cancer has now spread to his left lung. However, they are determined to remain positive and are keen not to rely entirely on the medical profession for help but want to do what they can for themselves, including changing their diet and using acupuncture. In spite of feeling weak and sick for periods of time, Gary wants to continue working. Initially he agrees to discuss their financial concerns, as Helen has also stopped working in a local shop to spend more time with Gary. They do not have any savings as 'we have always spent what we earn on the children'. Tearfully Gary concedes that he can cope with the cancer but he is more frightened about how they will manage financially if he has to stop working.

Gary was clearly experiencing a number of physical symptoms as a result of his condition and treatment. When he was offered the opportunity to discuss related issues, he established his own hierarchy of need, placing financial worry at the top. In an area of care where 'quality of life is not simply an aspect of concern but is the very raison d'être of every intervention' (Cohen and Mount 1992), the difficulties in measuring the concept in the palliative care population can be alleviated by agreeing with clients what is important to them. Financial worry has been shown to affect the quality of life of those with chronic and terminal illnesses (Pearlman and Uhlmann 1988; Cartwright 1992). Employment and higher socio-economic status has also been shown to provide the circumstances for better physical health and lower mortality following a bereavement (Martikainen and Valkonen 1998; Fitzpatrick and Bossé 2000). A dry mouth can all too easily remind patients of the reality of their illness but completing a benefit claim form can act as a painful confrontation with the diagnosis or the death that has occurred. It is vital that those working with these clients recognize the validity of this concern if their care is to be truly holistic. Moreover recognizing the possibility that money may be a source of concern is a necessary precursor to practitioners raising it as a legitimate area for discussion, intervention or referral on. The presence of physical needs does not necessarily relegate financial pain to a subsequent discussion, as Gary's situation demonstrates. Maslow's hierarchy of needs (1970) would suggest that individuals are motivated to meet their basic social needs before moving up to higher needs, including those of 'belonging', although this perspective and the needs stated might be regarded as portraying a particular cultural bias. This model has social needs competing at the same level as other physiological needs and there is no question that a patient's intractable physical pain will have to be addressed before other concerns can be considered, either by the patient or those in support. It would be unethical to discuss a benefit application with a patient distracted by a severe headache. However, the concept of 'total pain' also alerts us to the possibility of physical pain being exacerbated by causes other than chemical or physiological. Gary said that his worry about his family's financial situation did at times make his feelings of sickness seem worse and merely having the chance to talk through what his options were, 'took a big weight off my shoulders'.

Financial change

The state benefits system in the United Kingdom does offer some financial protection for the terminally ill and this country's collaborative approach to the provision of health and social care services should ensure that these services are free for those in the final stages of a terminal illness. Nevertheless, this group of people will not be immune from the costs of illness, such as increased heating and transport costs. Similar pressures are felt by those living with motor neurone disease and its more disabling features. The consequences of an illness and treatment may force many either to reduce their hours of work or stop completely. This is one of the most obvious causes of financial change for those living with advanced illness and the altered employment arrangements can be experienced equally by those in a caring role. It is vital not to forget that the 'bulk of community care is provided both free and freely within the immediate circles of those in receipt of it' (Drakeford 2001). Disability and carer benefits, if in payment, will help in ameliorating the loss of employment income but will rarely fully compensate this effect. Death brings with it huge implications for the surviving family members. One felt acutely by some is the financial consequence whereby the benefits claimed by the person who has died cease immediately and this comes at the same time as funeral expenses (Corden *et al.* 2002).

Following a diagnosis or bereavement, clients are faced with decisions about the future, their various relationships and have to cope with the emotions evoked. Finance-related problems are encountered alongside these other challenges and the former can be regarded by some as an insurmountable difficulty. These difficulties can include negotiations with an employer, knowing which state benefits are applicable and dealing with insurance companies. Many individuals will be able to deal with these issues without outside help. Professional resources are costly and in short supply; they should be offered to those in greatest need. This also reduces the risk of diminishing individuals' own strengths and resources through 'over-professionalism'. However, some clients will appreciate support in working their way through a maze of leaflets, applications, and bureaucratic language. Lack of awareness, inadequate specialist advice and insufficient knowledge amongst health and social care professionals have been found to present real barriers to benefit entitlement for cancer patients (Quinn 2002). Employment changes as a result of ill health may confront many with the prospect of claiming benefits for the first time though those already in receipt of entitlement may still require help in negotiating new rights or being made aware of their increased entitlement. The perceived stigmatizing effect of receiving benefits as well as a reluctance to feel dependent on a 'handout' or the fear of being seen as a fraud can prevent genuine claims being pursued (Costigan *et al.* 1999; Rowlingson *et al.* 1999; Age Concern 2001). Not having English as a first language will compound these barriers and women from ethnic minority communities have a particularly low take up of benefits (*www. disabilityalliance.org/r31.htm*).

Macmillan Cancer Relief commissioned a report to learn more about the problems encountered with benefits by people with cancer and converted it into an action plan for change (Quinn 2002). This user perspective can also be acted on by other services. As stated earlier, the level of help offered should be geared to the needs of the situation and this will range from providing a benefit form for a client to complete, to advocacy support when disputes arise and when clients feel physically or emotionally unable to proceed. This kind of high level and specialist assistance will need to be carried out by individuals with both the knowledge and time to see it through. Practitioners are required to be honest about their limits and have a clear understanding about whom to refer on to. These same practitioners, however, can respond in simpler ways to other benefit problems. Claim packs can be de-mystified for clients who perceive them as being too complicated to complete. Appropriate and clear reassurance about a person's right to benefit will enable some people suffering from misconceptions about their entitlement to apply. It is difficult to be precise about the monetary effect of the barriers to accessing benefits. Two sources put the estimates of benefit under claiming in the United Kingdom at between 10% and 60% (Dept of Social Security 1999; Quinn 2002), the higher figure relating to Disability Living Allowance (DLA) and Attendance Allowance (AA), crucial benefits for people with terminal illnesses in the United Kingdom. There will be a group of potential benefit claimants who will choose not to pursue their welfare rights even with sufficient information and support; this position has to be understood and accepted by those working with them. Nevertheless, there still appears to be a gap between entitlement and claiming which can be narrowed, with clients' permission, by practitioners working with those affected by terminal illness or the death of a family member.

The monetary aspect of financial pain is helped considerably by providing assistance for clients unaware of or tentative about approaching the benefits system. Empowering them by providing information and background support will be enough for many. Beyond this some individuals may appreciate and require help in liaising with organizations, which would be willing to be considerate of a person's ill health. Professional intervention with these organizations can often relieve clients' worries and circumvent any bureaucratic doubt regarding the genuineness of the situation. Practitioners have an advocacy and gatekeeping role in accessing financial help from charitable sources as applications usually have to be endorsed or submitted by a professional involved with the potential recipient. Information is available about charities operating at local and national levels (Harland and Griffiths 2000). These resources are far from comprehensive but they can be supplemented by an interested and creative worker who could act as a focal point for information within a team or service. Certainly the impact of these grants should not be underestimated either in financial terms or in relation to the need they can address.

A psychological component

Financial pain is a multi-faceted concept that is not confined to managing on a low income and may be experienced by those living with a limited prognosis or following the death of someone close to them. It is not the exclusive domain of individuals or families whose low socio-economic status pre-existed the diagnosis. Financial pain is based on the universality of loss and change in their various guises; even those from a financially stable background can be affected by the social implications serious illness and death bring. In the United Kingdom, homeowners with a mortgage have been traditionally perceived as financially secure and yet they can often face greater uncertainty if their ill health results in them claiming the appropriate means-tested benefit, Income Support. The allowance for housing costs attached to this benefit is delayed for those with a mortgage whereas those in rented accommodation generally receive financial assistance immediately. Whilst families already on a low income may feel living with the uncertainty of serious illness adds to the difficulties they face, a high earning bank manager may be equally distressed by being forced to leave his job and consider using savings to pay for private care. Those working with these situations should be mindful of the uniqueness of the experience for the families and individuals involved and not apply absolute measures of poverty or attempt to arrange a hierarchy of social need on their caseload; financial pain is a relative concept.

Financial pain also has other elements at various levels of visibility. Returning to the earlier case example, Gary did eventually agree to have help in applying for DLA but not until after a great deal of deliberation. During this consideration he reflected tearfully on how he had always hoped to provide for his family by working, as his father had done for him and his siblings. He admitted that his pride had not allowed him to pursue what might be rightfully his to claim and he was worried that embarking on a dependency on state benefits would represent a capitulation to the illness. For Gary and many others, financial change, including both the reduction of income and restructuring of their income profile, denotes parallel losses. The 'secondary stressors' associated with job loss, which will be different from person to person can be expected to incorporate changes to identity, self esteem, social support, and control (Price *et al.* 1998). Gary's role as provider for his family had been severely challenged by his ill health. He tearfully declared to his wife that he felt he had let her and the children down, as well as himself, when he ultimately reduced his working hours. Older people who develop serious illness after retirement can also experience a range of feelings as a result of serious illness or bereavement and their financial consequences. Frustration can occur at learning of their ill health at a time when they had planned so much and saved over a long period to enable them to do it or anger about using their monetary legacy to pay for institutional care. Certainly, those in a higher income group may have better material means to cope with their illness but it will probably be a different kind of life from the one expected.

Seeing the potential for the emotional in the practical and vice versa is a core skill of good psychosocial palliative care; it is also at the heart of what is meant by financial pain. The philosophy of integrating 'the purely psychological and the practical as they touch people's social lives' (Oliviere 2001) has been identified with social work practice with the dying and bereaved by others (Currer 2001; Small 2001). The wider multi-disciplinary team also needs to recognize this dynamic to ensure a holistic approach to care. Nurses in the United Kingdom often have the responsibility of assisting patients with claims for DLA and AA in palliative care services. It will often be appropriate to make these claims under Special Rules, a process specifically introduced to speed up the receipt of benefit so that patients living with a limited prognosis are not disadvantaged by relatively slow decision-making processes (Nosowska 2003). The financial gain of a successful claim for DLA and AA under Special Rules is not inconsiderable. Creating a partnership with clients and working with what is permissible is a clear way of 'handing back as much control as possible to the person whose body is out of control' (Oliviere *et al.* 1998). Discussing Gary and Helen's approach to their illness, including their need to look for complementary treatments, indicated the importance of control as a way of coping. They were left with information about his entitlement to DLA so that his eventual decision to proceed with an application was paced around their need for time to consider their options and to discuss the emotional impact of the decision, as a couple and with the social worker.

In spite of the potential for an emotional layer to financial concerns, they can often prove a safe starting point for engagement with a health professional. Referrals for assistance with financial matters will regularly, though not always, lead to conversations about other concerns. This does not happen by chance but as a result of the practitioner demonstrating sensitivity and good communication skills in one area which the clients have assumed would be applied to other worries. With limited prognoses, having enough time to discuss certain financial issues can be a concern for both families and practitioners. Within the boundaries of patient and family choice it can be helpful for a worker to be pro-active in creating opportunities for discussion about scenarios seemingly too painful to raise. Asking a couple living with a terminal illness whether they have any financial concerns about the future can empower some to explore doubts about funeral costs and the making of a will.

Intrinsic to palliative care is equal respect for the needs of carers alongside the patients'. Couples sometimes struggle to acknowledge and accept their differing social and information needs. Professionals will be challenged to work in these situations also. Being clear about the differences and the normality of this can be reassuring. Providing support individually after proper joint agreement about this way of working will help some relationships. Helen was able to discuss openly with Gary how she preferred not to go to work at present as she found it hard to respond to the concerned enquiries from her colleagues about her husband. She was also keen to apply for a Carer's Allowance as soon as possible rather than take the time Gary had needed. Once again discussions about finances in the future, individually or jointly, may initially provide the means for explaining entitlement but will at times also lead to concerns about the emotional impact of living alone or as a single parent. When working with the financial needs of the recently bereaved, it is vital that feelings evoked about changes to status or role have an opportunity to be shared. The forms to be completed at this time can painfully face an individual with their new identity as a widow or bereaved parent. If unchecked and unsupported these feelings can both create a barrier to claiming the benefit and leave the bereaved person isolated and confused.

Practice and service implications

Practice and services are directly influenced by the values of individual workers and the organization. For example, nurses' attitudes towards tissue donation have been shown to impact on family decisions (Wells and Sque 2002). In relation to financial issues, more disconcerting is Walker and Walker's belief that social workers' regular exposure to clients in poverty dulls their recognition of it and its discriminating implications (1998).

Social work's familiarity with the universality of loss equips it to practise in palliative care (Currer 2000). The profession also has a strong tradition of providing welfare rights advice (Payne 2002) and this sits comfortably with its commitment to social justice and anti-discriminatory practice. In the United Kingdom, the Association of Hospice and Specialist Palliative Care Social Workers has drawn on this tradition stating that the social work task includes assessing a 'patient's, family's and carer's ... financial needs' and providing 'information and advocacy regarding DSS (Department of Social Security) benefits and charitable help' (AHSPCSW 2000). This strong link with social care may have been the reason why cancer patients preferred the inclusion of a social worker in local Macmillan teams as an effective means of providing benefits advice (Quinn 2002). This research also found that service users valued the idea of health professionals undertaking welfare rights training, though interestingly, this was less popular with the practitioners questioned. Social workers are not part of every palliative care team and it is apparent that social workers in this field intervene with financial needs to varying degrees. Other ways of providing welfare rights advice exist, such as the presence of specialist welfare officers (Bechelet and Boultwood 2001). In the absence of a consensus about the need for social work as an essential part of palliative care multi-disciplinary teams or uniformity about their role where they are present, services will need to think creatively about their response to financial pain.

Table 11.1 Reviewing commitment to financial pain at organizational, systems, and practitioner levels

Response level	Key questions
Organization Philosophy	◆ Do the service aims and objectives reflect the diversity of need for clients?
	◆ Is financial need included in the philosophy of care for clients?
	◆ Is financial need regarded as requiring both a generalist and specialist response?
Structure	◆ Is the team multi-professional with someone responsible for clients' financial needs and/or is there a clear access point for specialist financial advice from another agency?
	◆ Is this support available for the bereaved?
	◆ Do links with external professionals/agencies need to be developed to enhance the provision of financial care?

(Continued)

Table 11.1 (continued) Reviewing commitment to financial pain at organizational, systems, and practitioner levels

Response level	Key questions
Training	◆ Is financial pain and basic benefit entitlement included in training for all clinical staff?
	◆ How is specialist knowledge or skill level assessed and updated?
	◆ Does the bereavement service include financial awareness as part of training?
Systems Assessment	Are financial concerns incorporated in initial assessment, review and bereavement risk/needs assessment forms?
	◆ Are there prompts on this documentation to facilitate assessment of financial need?
	◆ Do all professionals contribute to and access assessment documentation?
	◆ How are clients' views on financial concerns assessed?
Communication & Information	◆ Is there information available for clients about financial help? Is it available in different formats/languages? How often is it reviewed?
	◆ What are the systems for making specialist referral for clients in financial need?
	◆ Does a focal point for local/national resources exist within the service?
Practitioner Knowledge	◆ What is the knowledge level of the practitioner in relation to financial needs?
	◆ Do all practitioners have an understanding of essential welfare rights information?
	◆ Does the practitioner know when, whom, and how to refer for specialist financial advice?
Attitude	◆ How does the practitioner view financial need as a potential concern for clients?
	◆ How may the individual's practice discriminate against financial needs?
	◆ How and with whom does the practitioner discuss how their practice is influenced by their own values?

Table 11.1 presumes a wide variation of service models which will address financial pain in clients' lives and these will vary in accordance with personnel available on the team and local resources. This way of reviewing a service is also predicated on certain assumptions. Firstly, services and individuals within them are willing and have the means to review their provision of care. Secondly, good psychosocial care is the responsibility of all professionals working with clients and this includes an ability, at a basic level, to work with financial needs. This is essential when working with individuals and families whose needs intertwine and 'do not come in neat discrete boxes with discrete professional labels' (Monroe 1998). Thirdly, financial pain is not expected to gain special but equal treatment by services and workers. Initially, measures may need to be taken to positively promote its profile where it has not previously received appropriate consideration. Finally, the table can be used wholesale by multi-professional, specialist palliative care teams or selectively by those individuals, whether team based or not, providing palliative care as part of their duties (e.g. General Practitioners, Intensive Therapy Unit staff, and community nurses).

Conclusion

Those working with the dying and bereaved will frequently encounter families living in financial need. For many of these families their poverty will have pre-dated their diagnosis or bereavement and it is incumbent upon professionals to understand the discrimination and disadvantage they will have experienced in their lives. Only then will practitioners be able to work effectively with the full extent and complexity of their loss during their illness or bereavement (Bevan 2002). Financial pain has been introduced as a concept which recognizes the totality of need for those coming into contact with palliative care agencies and is based on the known changes these individuals experience to income and other related visible issues, including employment and housing. Financial pain can be felt by those already living on a low income which is exacerbated by ill health or the death of a family member, but it is also a relevant need for those people whose material circumstances are significantly altered by either experience. This is in part due to a belief in the uniqueness of each individual's experience. It is also explained by the multi-dimensional nature of financial pain which asserts an unquestionable relationship between the visible losses mentioned and the less obvious changes to status, self-esteem, and relationships.

The paucity of research into the importance and ramifications of financial need for the dying and bereaved may well reflect a parallel profile for financial pain in palliative care services. These services and professionals within them need to examine the way they are structured and practise as a way of ensuring that more than lip service is paid to the principle of 'total care for total pain' (Saunders 1993). If this does not happen then these care providers are in danger of adding discrimination and insensitivity to existing disadvantage and loss.

References

Age Concern (2001) *Benefit Take Up and Older People*. Policy paper ref. 0101. Age Concern, England.

Association of Hospice and Specialist Palliative Care Social Workers (2000) *Members' Handbook*.

Bechelet L and Boultwood L (2001) Welfare and benefit issues affecting people with terminal illness. *Palliative Care Today* **X**(1):10–11.

Bevan D (2002) Poverty and deprivation. In Thompson N (ed.) *Loss and Grief: a Guide for Human Services Practitioners*, pp. 93–107. Palgrave, Hants.

Blane D, Bartley M, and Davey Smith G (1998) Making sense of socio-economic health equalities. In Field D and Taylor S (ed.) *Sociological Perspectives on Health, Illness and Health Care*, pp. 79–96. Blackwell Science, Oxford.

Cartwright A (1992) Social class differences in health and care in the year before death. *Journal of Epidemiology and Community Health* **46**:54–7.

Clark D and Seymour J (1999) *Reflections on Palliative Care*. Open University Press, Buckingham.

Cohen SR and Mount BM (1992) Quality of life in terminal illness: defining and measuring subjective well-being in the dying. *Journal of Palliative Care* **8**(3):40–5.

Corden A, Sloper P, and Sainsbury R (2002) Financial effects for families after the death of a disabled or chronically ill child: a neglected dimension of bereavement. *Child: Care, Health and Development* **28**(3):199–204.

Costigan P, Finch H, Jackson B, Legard R, and Ritchie J (1999) Overcoming barriers: older people and income support. *Dept of Social Security*.

Currer C (2001) *Responding to Grief: Dying, Bereavement and Social Care*. Palgrave, Hants.

Drakeford M (2001) Poverty and the social services. In Bytheway B, Bacigalupo V, Bornat J, Johnson J, and Spurr S (ed.) *Understanding Care, Welfare and Community: A Reader*, pp. 29–37. Routledge, London.

Dept of Social Security (1999) *Social Security Departmental Report. The Government Expenditure Plans* 21.4.99.

Ferriss AL (2002) Does material well-being affect non-material well-being? *Social Indicators Research* **60**:275–80.

Field D (2000) *What Do We Mean By 'Psychosocial'?* Briefing Paper no. 4. National Council for Hospice and Specialist Palliative Care Services, London.

Fitzpatrick TR and Bossé R (2000) Employment and health among older bereaved men in the normative aging study: one year and three years following a bereavement event. *Social Work in Health Care* 32(2):41–60.

Gallagher D (2002) *Financial Pain: A Study of the Finance Related Concerns of Cancer Patients and Their Partners Receiving Palliative Care.* MSc dissertation, Southampton University (Unpublished).

Harland S and Griffiths D (2000) *A Guide to Grants for Individuals in Need.* Directory of Social Change, London.

Hunt R (1997) Place of death of cancer patients. *Progress in Palliative Care* 5(6): 238–42.

Landau R (1995) Locus of control and socio-economic status: does locus of control reflect real resources and opportunities or personal coping abilities? *Social Science and Medicine*, 41(11):1499–1505.

Martikainen P and Valkonen T (1998) Do education and income buffer the effects of death of spouse on mortality? *Epidemiology* 9(5):530–3.

Maslow AH (1970) *Motivation and personality*, (2nd edn). Harper and Row, New York.

Monroe B (1998) Social work in palliative care. In Doyle D, Hanks G, and MacDonald N (ed.) *Oxford Textbook of Palliative Medicine* Oxford, OUP.

National Council for Hospice and Specialist Palliative Care Services (2001) *Building on success: strategic agenda for 2001–2004.* National Council, London.

NHS (2000) The NHS cancer plan: a plan for investment, a plan for reform. Dept of Health.

Nosowska G (2003) Fatal delay. *Community Care* 30: Jan – 5 Feb, 2003, 40.

Oliviere D (2001) The social worker in palliative care—the 'eccentric' role. *Progress in Palliative Care* 9:237–41.

Oliviere D, Hargreaves R, and Monroe B (1998) *Good Practices in Palliative Care: A Psychosocial Perspective.* Ashgate, Aldershot.

Parkes CM (1990) Risk factors in bereavement: implications for the prevention and treatment of pathologic grief. *Psychiatric Annals*, 20:6, 308–13.

Payne M (2002) Balancing the equation. *Professional Social Work*, January 2002, 12–3.

Pearlman RA and Uhlmann RF (1988) Quality of life in chronic diseases: perceptions of elderly patients. *Journal of Gerontology* 43(2) M25–30.

Pettinger N (1999) Richly deserving. *Health Service Journal* 9 Sept. 99:20–1.

Price RH, Friedland DS, and Vinokur AD (1998) Job loss: hard times and eroded identity. In Harvey JH (ed.) *Perspectives On Loss—a Sourcebook.* Brunner/Mazel, USA.

Quinn A (2002) *Macmillan Cancer Relief Study into Benefits Advice for People with Cancer*. MCR, London.

Relf M (2000) *The Effectiveness of Volunteer Bereavement Care: an Evaluation of a Palliative Care Bereavement Service*. PhD Thesis, Goldsmith College, London (Unpublished).

Rowlingson K with Black P, Harrington A, and Merrin W (1999) *A Balancing Act: Surviving the Risk Society*. NACAB, London.

Saunders C (1993) Introduction—'history and challenge'. In Saunders C and Sykes N (ed.) *The Management of Terminal Malignant Disease* (3rd edn), pp. 11–14. Hodder and Stoughton, London.

Sheldon F (2003) Social impact of advanced metastatic cancer. In Lloyd-Williams M (ed.) *Psychosocial Issues in Palliative Care*. OUP, Oxford.

Small N (2001) Social work and palliative care. *British Journal of Social Work* 31:961–71.

Soothill K, Morris SM, Harman J, Francis B, Thomas C, *et al.* (2001*a*) The significant unmet needs of cancer patients: probing psychosocial concerns. *Supportive Care in Cancer* 9:597–605.

Soothill K, Morris SM, Harman JC, Francis B, Thomas C, *et al.* (2001*b*) Informal carers of cancer patients: what are their unmet psychosocial needs? *Health and Social Care in the Community* 9(6):464–75.

Walker C and Walker A (1998) Social work and society. In Adams RL, Dominelli L, and Payne M (ed.) *Social Work: Themes, Issues and Critical Debates*. Palgrave, London.

Wells J and Sque M (2002) 'Living choice': the commitment to tissue donation in palliative care. *International Journal of Palliative Nursing* 8:22–7.

Wright EP, Kiely MA, Lynch P, Cull A, and Selby PJ (2002) Social problems in oncology. *British Journal of Cancer* 87:1099–104.

Wyatt GK, Friedman L, Given CW, and Given BA. (1999) A profile of bereaved caregivers following provision of terminal care. *Journal of Palliative Care* 15(1):13–25.

12

Carers and caregivers

Sheila Payne

Introduction

In this chapter I am going to address a series of questions about a group of people who are crucially important in the lives of people facing the end of life, yet they are often relegated in health and social care textbooks and even policy documents, to a marginal status. These people are the families and friends of those who are ill and who may or may not identify themselves with the terms carer or caregiver. I will discuss the impact of disease and illness upon those people who are in close relationships with the ill person. Human beings are social animals, embedded within social systems, kinship networks, and cultural groups. Families, friends, and cultural groups are affected by life-threatening illness and the potential loss of a person. Indeed, the lack of such networks is potentially problematic especially near the end of life. For example, the situation for those without such close relationships is very difficult perhaps because they have lived to late old age, moved to new countries like refugees and asylum seekers, or experienced other types of social exclusion such as homelessness or imprisonment. For these people, established social support and social networks are not readily available in the period before death.

This chapter will start by considering who becomes a carer. The term 'carer' is attributed by health and social care workers to the main person responsible for the ill person but is it understood and used in the same way by family and friends? The following section explores what it is that carers actually do. I wish to challenge the accepted assumption that caregiving is primarily involved with physical tasks which are *done for* the ill person and therefore are burdensome. I will consider the evidence which suggests that carers are frequently involved in psychological and social care (Payne and

Ellis-Hill 2001). Moreover, these other types of care are often hidden and unacknowledged, but are very demanding.

Most caregiving relationships are highly complex because they are built upon long shared histories (for example in marriage) and mutually agreed, or at least taken-for-granted ways of relating which may be challenged by the changes brought about by advanced illness such as physical deterioration or financial dependency. Moreover, the reciprocal nature of relationships within family care giving, means that it is very difficult for carers to prioritise their own needs above those of the patient. This will provide the context for considering different types of relationships between service providers and carers. Many health and social care workers assume that there is a single, main carer but this may not be the case. Family members may evolve different roles in supporting the ill person and their needs may differ over time. I will examine the extent to which health and social care workers establish effective communication channels which may well need to differ between families and within families over time.

In the remainder of the chapter, the evidence about the efficacy of interventions to support carers, such as information provision, support groups and respite care will be discussed. While there is a wealth of literature on carers, especially those caring for older people and children, much less research has focused on the needs of those caring for people near the end of life. Does this matter? Is research on carers transferable across different types of care? The chapter ends by considering these questions.

Who are carers?

According to the General Household Survey conducted in 2000, there are approximately seven million carers in the UK (Maher and Green 2002). The majority of carers provide care for those with chronic illness, disabilities, and for frail older people. It is difficult to estimate the number of those providing care for a person nearing the end of life, as much will depend upon the definition of palliative care used and whether the remit extends to those with chronic life limiting diseases such as dementia, heart failure, and end-stage renal disease. However, the evidence suggests that greater numbers of people provide care at some point in their lives than ten years ago. More women (approximately 3.9 million) than men (2.9 million) provide care (Maher and Green 2002). Data from the General Household Survey, indicated that the majority of carers were middle aged (between 45–64 years) but increasingly older people over 65 years, are involved in caring both for their spouse and parents who may now live into late old age (over 85 years). In palliative care, there is more likely to be within genera-tional than cross-generational care giving, which is different from other types of caring. There is little data on the extent to which children provide care but it has been estimated that approximately 51,000 young people under 16 years, are involved in care for other ill or disabled family mem-bers but only a small number of whom are dying (Walker 1996). Segal and Simkins (1993) have documented the impact on children of being involving in providing care for parents with chronic neurological conditions such as multiple sclerosis.

Lay people who take on unpaid caring roles in relation to a person fac-ing the end of life are usually defined as carers or care-givers. These people are usually the family members or relatives but changing social patterns such as divorce, geographical mobility, increased longevity and declining birth rates, may mean that for some people, friends, neighbours, or employed care workers (for example, for older people living in care homes) may provide more significant and meaningful relationships than distant kin. It should not be assumed that all family members may be able or wish to take on a caring role.

The definition of 'family' is potentially problematic because it is neces-sary to include those people who share biological, social, or legal ties. It also includes those related by continuing heterosexual and same sex relation-ships and extended family relationships and broader culturally recognized social groups either through birth, adoption, or legal contract (marriage). What constitutes a 'family' may vary between cultures, from a dyad (for example, a mother and child) to a multigenerational dynasty. Perhaps a defining feature of a family is the sense of enduring emotional and social bonds experienced by members. Whatever the definitional problems with the term 'family', it should be acknowledged that families are dynamic social structures. Families change over time as members are added through mar-riage, birth, and adoption and lost through death and in some cultures following marriage. There are role expectations, responsibilities, and com-mitments which are often related to economic provision, childbearing and child raising activities and in some cultures these roles may be defined by gender. Theories tend to describe family relationships in terms of complex systems of reciprocal demands and support.

Social changes in Western countries have impacted upon family structures and the availability of family members to fulfil caring roles. These changes include: increasing divorce and separation, where individuals through a life time may experience a series of marital or partnership relationships and their children a series of family relationships with step-parenting and step siblings becoming common. Increased longevity may result in greater numbers of people enjoying being grand or great grand parents but also increasing the possibility of experiencing the loss of, or distancing from, family members in late old age. In many countries there is a declining birth rate with some people remaining childless (approximately 10% of women in the UK) and family size has declined to one or two children per partnership. This reduces the potential number of people related by kinship who may be available to offer care near the end of life. Economic pressures for two incomes combined with other factors have increased female employment rates, while male employment patterns have become less stable with greater geographical mobility and more part-time working.

There are certain groups in society who may be less likely to have close family ties. Perhaps the most obvious are those people who have rejected, or been rejected by their families. It is important to remember that not all families are mutually supportive or beneficial to their members. As well as being supportive, families may also be characterized by abusive, exploitative, or threatening relationships. For individuals in these situations, families may not contribute to their welfare. Older people, especially those in late old age are an increasing proportion of the population in many developed countries. These people may be vulnerable to social isolation as families become dispersed and friends die. Approximately a fifth of all people over 85 years in the UK die in residential or nursing homes. These older people may have family members but they may also develop close emotional and social relationships with their peers in care homes and with care staff. There may be socially disadvantaged or socially excluded people such as refugees, homeless people, and prisoners, who may not have access to families or friends to support them during times of crisis.

What do carers do?

Being a carer is a social relationship that can only be undertaken in the context of another person, even if that person rejects the carer or is reluctant to be cared for. Research undertaken with older people indicates that many of them are fearful of becoming dependent upon family members and do not wish to 'burden' their adult children (Seymour *et al.* 2002). So becoming a carer and becoming a cared for person, are social roles for which many people experience some ambivalence (see Box 1). On the one hand, providing care is challenging and may impact negatively upon the care provider, it may also be rewarding and enjoyable, developing and enhancing existing social and familial bonds. In addition, carers may derive social approval and increased self esteem in knowing they have done all they can for their loved one. This may reduce feelings of guilt and distress during bereavement.

Box 1 The impact of caring upon carers

Negative consequences
Physical health
Psychological health
Social isolation
Financial demands

Positive consequences
Closer relationship
Expression of love and affection
Fulfilment of duty
Earning the respect of others

Much of the early research on carers emphasized the domestic and personal care tasks which were performed, this lead to a picture of carers being physically burdened by the labour of caring which has been critiqued by Nolan (2001). There are a number of ways to conceptualize and categorize caring. Drawing on the work of Nolan *et al.* (1995) who built upon the earlier formulations of Bowers (1987), the following offers one way to conceptualize types of caring:

- Anticipatory care
- Preventative care
- Supervisory care
- Instrumental care
- Protective care
- Preservative care
- (Re)constructive care
- Reciprocal care.

While lists may not be very helpful in a practical sense because types of care may overlap considerably, they are useful in highlighting 'hidden' elements of caring. For example, in caring for a person near the end of life, the carer may spend time in the early stages, when there are relatively few physical problems, anticipating and planning for deterioration in physical abilities. They may spend time supporting the person emotionally, managing interactions with other family members, containing family distress and anxiety. Carers may describe this type of care as 'being strong', 'being there' or 'being positive'. The emotional labour of care giving is largely unacknowledged by professionals and carers may not even recognize these activities as 'care work'. But in the context of life-threatening illness, carers typically manage the feelings of patients, manage the feelings of other family members and friends and manage their own feelings. Taken-for-granted social rules mean that generally carers put the patient first and hide or minimize their own feelings. While carers may be concerned about some of the same issues as the ill person, they may also be worried about their own future; how they will cope with the death and bereavement, and have financial worries which may be difficult to share with the ill person.

In an ethnographic study conducted in The Netherlands (The 2002), spouses of patients with lung cancer spent many hours accompanying their relatives to cancer clinics and helped them as advocates and as mediators in acquiring information from health care staff. It may only be during the later stages of the illness, that physical caring such as assistance with washing, toileting, and feeding become necessary. At this stage, family carers may take on responsibility for nursing tasks such as giving medication, cleaning a urinary catheter, or changing stoma bags. Smith (2001) found, in a series of detailed case studies of carers of palliative care patients at home, that providing personal and nursing care tended to alter the nature of relationships and was difficult to manage for both parties. Moreover, some carers were concerned that they would not perform the tasks correctly and some cared for people were uncomfortable with intimate care tasks such as bathing being undertaken by family members especially those of a different gender. For example, it may be difficult for a daughter to perform personal care for her father or grandfather. In these situations, some patients and carers prefer care to be undertaken by paid health or social care workers.

In addition to providing care for the ill person, carers often take on additional responsibilities in managing the home, family finances, childcare, and care of other dependents such as older relatives. In a recent study of carers of those with cancer (Thomas *et al.* 2002), 21% of carers were already carers before the cancer diagnosis. It is important not to assume that the terminally ill person is the only responsibility that the carer has. There may be a reallocation of care tasks for example a father may take on more childcare activities from his ill wife, and there may be creation of new tasks related to the care of the ill person. These may be new roles for the person who has to manage the demands of the ill person with on-going family demands. The diagnosis of a terminal condition in a family member may precipitate major role transitions for all family members. For example, older children may have to take on domestic tasks or caring for younger siblings. Barnard *et al.* (2000) provide an account of a cancer patient called Albert Hoffer, who was the primary carer for his wife who had had a stroke. They described the complex caring arrangements made by family members and professional workers in supporting this couple both of whom were ill. This highlights another issue, in that carers, especially older carers, may have health problems and disabilities which may be exacerbated or be caused by their care giving activities, such as back pain.

Not all care-giving relationships are supportive and recent research has started to identify problematic aspects. Rook and Pietromonaco (1987) highlighted four unsupportive factors:

- ineffective help
- excessive help that increased recipient dependence
- unwanted or unpleasant interactions
- encouragement of unhealthy behaviours.

Conflict may be experienced in all families but in families where conflict is unresolved, long standing or violent, the establishment of caring relationships for an ill person is especially problematic. Conflict may be more intense in small kinship networks where increasingly heavy demands are placed upon relatively few people compared to larger more diverse social networks where there are more resources for people to draw upon and the potential for overloading each individual is less. This has implications for health and social care practitioners working with certain groups of people such as those with few social contacts (e.g. people who have moved to a new area to retire), those who are alienated from others because of poor social skills, alcohol or substance abuse, or those living in socially disadvantaged communities.

In a study conducted in Canada by Neufeld and Harrison (2003) with carers of people with dementia, two main categories of non-support were identified.

Unmet expectations

- unfulfilled or missing offers
- unmet expectations for social interactions
- mismatched aid
- incompetence.

Negative interactions

- ◆ disparaging comments
- ◆ conflict in appraisal of the care recipient's health status
- ◆ criticism
- ◆ spillover of conflict from other issues.

This study provides a useful reminder that social support may function in undesirable as well as desirable ways. Moreover, both aspects may be experienced during the course of care giving relationships. Research from Israel provides evidence from carers of those with dementia that their feelings of competence and satisfaction with their role of carer can co-exist with feelings of burden (Greenberger and Litwin 2003). Both the last two cited studies have been drawn from the experience of care giving to those with dementia. Typically the illness trajectory in dementia is more prolonged than some other types of care giving such as for those with cancer and heart failure.

What is the nature of carers' relationships with service providers?

In the past it was regarded as normal for patients to be separated from their relatives and friends on entry into hospital, even children were limited in their contact with parents. Visiting by relatives and friends was restricted both in time and numbers of people (usually two to a bed). The visiting times were organized for the benefit of the institution, rather than allowing easy access for relatives, and were usually strictly controlled by nursing staff. Hawker (1983) in an ethnographic account of nurses' interactions with patients' relatives, identified a range of strategies used by nurses to discourage and limit their contact with questioning relatives such as the legitimate gait—a purposeful and 'busy' walking style on the ward, with careful avoidance of eye-contact. Relatives were typically regarded as 'in the way' and a nuisance by medical and nursing staff. Latterly relatives, relabelled as 'carers', have been regarded as participants in delivering care. In some post stroke care services, for example, it is now common for professionals to invite carers to be involved in discharge planning and rehabilitation (Low et al. 1999). There is recognition that carers need skills and knowledge to deliver care. There is also recognition that they should also be willing and informed when making the decision to take up the role of carer. But in reality many relatives take up the care-giver role either by default, as no-one else is available to provide care, or at a time of crisis. It may then be very difficult to relinquish these tasks. Research by Smith (2001) found that community nurses, general practitioners, and specialist palliative care practitioners largely assumed that relatives would become carers of palliative care patients.

The 'voices' of carers

It is only recently that patients and carers have been invited to contribute directly to national debates on health and social care or become involved in the planning and delivery of services and contribute to the design and conduct of research in health care (The National Cancer Alliance 1996; Department of Health 1999/2000; Crawford *et al.* 2002). Even within these new 'user involvement' policies, carers tend to be regarded as proxies for patients too ill or otherwise unable to articulate their own views rather than as having a mandate to speak about their own concerns. The authors of The National Cancer Alliance (1996) reported that 'even when carers were alone together in carers' groups, it proved quite difficult to persuade carers to speak about their own needs'. Evidence from this study and a large survey of 58644 cancer patients (Department of Health 1999/2000) indicated that carers were marginalized during medical consultations, sometimes at the wishes of patients themselves. For example, 42% of cancer patients reported that family and friends were involved in their out-patient care or treatment discussions but 31% were not at the request of patients, while 19% had no carer. Carers are often coping in relative isolation and managing their role with relatively little first-hand information and even less emotional support directed towards their needs. The following excerpt from the husband of a person with Hodgkin's disease illustrates this:

> Everybody that phoned up always wanted to know, how's X? Nobody asked about me, which I just accepted as normal. I was left to cope with it as best I could. (The National Cancer Alliance 1996)

In an attempt to highlight the needs and views of carers, CancerVOICES, a national network of cancer service users, has been established. This recent initiative seeks to empower patients and carers to be more proactive in influencing services and health care policies in the UK. They provide skills training and support service users in a range of ways, often working through cancer networks. While these initiatives are to be welcomed, careful thought needs to be given to ensure that they are tailored to the unique circumstances of palliative care, where patients have advanced disease and are likely to be physically frail with high levels of symptom burden, and carers may be facing difficult physical and psychological challenges as the patients' health deteriorates (Gott *et al.* 2002).

How do carers and service providers communicate?

A number of terms are used to describe the same group of people (see Box 2) but each term positions them in a different type of social relationship with health and social care workers as noted above.

Box 2 Terms used to describe people associated with the ill person

- Carers
- Care givers
- Care takers
- Informal carers
- Companions
- Relatives
- Family
- Friends
- Significant others
- Next of kin
- Visitors

Twigg and Atkin (1994) have highlighted the ambiguous position occupied by carers in relation to their interactions with service providers. They proposed four theoretical models and a further one was added by Nolan *et al.* (1995), which typified the response of services to carers.

Carers as resources

Twigg and Atkin (1994) suggest that this model is the taken for granted assumption of most services. From this position, relatives and especially spouses are seen as automatically available to care for the dependent person. Carers are regarded as appendages to the client or patient who is regarded as the 'proper' focus of attention of the professional. There is no onus on professionals to consider the wishes or needs of carers. Within the context of palliative care, it may be taken to imply that the patients' wishes, for example, for a home death, should be prioritized over all other considerations. Nolan *et al.* (1996) have argued that this way of regarding carers is both morally and ethically indefensible.

Carers as co-workers

An alternative model is to regard the carer as a joint worker with professionals in delivering optimal care for the benefit of the patient. While this acknowledges the position of the carer within the enterprise of care, it makes assumptions that there are agreed aims and strategies, for achieving desired outcomes. Thus professional support and services may be directed at enabling carers to continue to provide care, when this might be detrimental to the carer's own health and welfare.

Carers as co-clients

This model explicitly acknowledges that the carer is an individual within his/her own right and has needs, wishes, and roles, which extend beyond the caring role. In the UK, legislation has recognized that carers have rights to individual assessments. However, it is still potentially pathologizing as it proposes that carers are in need of professional services.

The superseded carer

This category of carer arises in two ways according to Twigg and Atkin (1994). Firstly, as a recognition that for some people remaining in a caring relationship is potentially disempowering. For example, young adults with chronic illnesses such as cystic fibrosis who are now increasingly living into their 20s and 30s, may wish to separate themselves from the vigilance and care of their parents (Small and Rhodes 2000). For these parents, it may be a difficult task to step back from active engagement in their off-springs' lives, especially when at the time of diagnosis the child was probably anticipated to have a limited prognosis. Secondly, the superseded carer model refers to those people who have decided to relinquish the role of carer. While this is generally thought to apply to carers of older people who decide that institutional care is the preferred option, it may also have parallels in palliative care when the burden of caring or acute problems with symptom control mean that admission to in-patient care is accepted (Hinton 1994*a*, *b*).

Carer as expert

In an addition to Twigg and Atkin (1994)s typology of carers, Nolan *et al.* (1995) proposed that carers should be regarded as 'experts' in the care of their dependent person. They have identified that carers build up considerable expertise in the best way to deal with the unique features of their cared for person, for example, how best to make them comfortable, how to interpret signs of distress and pain in aphasic people. Within this conceptualization, two types of knowledge are legitimized; the individual lived experience of 'knowing' a person over many years (the carer's knowledge) and the generalized 'professional' knowledge of service providers. Each person has a source of knowledge, which could potentially contribute to the welfare of the dependent person. However, power and knowledge differentials within the professional–carer relationship may mean that there may not be mutual respect for each other's contribution. In particular, carers may be reluctant to challenge professionals' ways of working, especially when the cared for person is admitted to hospital or other institution such as a nursing home, where professional patterns of working are dominant.

What interventions are available for carers and how supportive are they?

Having identified that carers for people requiring palliative care have high levels of need, this section considers the evidence on the efficacy of the interventions designed to respond to these needs. A systematic review of interventions for carers indicated there was no conclusive evidence of the efficacy or cost effectiveness of any one type of intervention compared to others (Harding and Higginson 2003). The authors were critical of the research that was available because it tended to be descriptive and relied on small samples. However, they acknowledged the difficulty in designing studies, using methods such as randomized controlled trials because of the complexity and individual nature of the interventions required by different carers. Similar conclusions were made in relation to interventions for carers supporting people following a stroke (Low *et al.* 1999). A number of interventions have been developed to assist carers. These can be broadly grouped into three categories:

- – Provision of information and education,
- – Provision of support either in groups or one-to-one counselling,
- – Respite.

Provision of information and education

According to Harding and Higginson (2003) provision of information and education is the most common type of intervention delivered to carers.

This is based on the assumption that carers have a deficit of knowledge and skills, which health and social care workers can supply. It is also based on the assumption that increasing knowledge and providing information is helpful and empowering, rather than anxiety provoking and potentially confusing. Most information is provided in face-to-face interactions with health and social care workers and these are often highly valued because they can be directed to the specific concerns and circumstances of each carer. But time pressures on health and social care workers, lack of communication skills in both parties and concerns about patient confidentially may inhibit exchange of information. Other common means of supplying information is in written formats or using information technology. Dixon-Woods (2001) has been critical of the way written information leaflets have been shaped by a view that patients and carers need education about the medical aspects of the disease. Written information is often produced by health professionals and provides information about medical aspects of care, rather than experiential aspects which may only be known by fellow patients and carers. She argues that this has given rise to leaflets written in simplistic language which fails to capture the debate and ambivalence around treatment and care options. Information leaflets tend to concentrate on addressing issues of concern to the patient and their care, rather than acknowledging the separate concerns and needs of carers. Thus patients and carers tend to be critical of the general and often bland, written information provided by professionals. In another health care arena, the disability rights lobby have challenged the rights of others to produce information on their behalf. In the future, it may be more appropriate for patients and carers to produce their own information resources, just as they have started to do in the context of Internet websites and discussion groups.

Provision of support either in groups or one-to-one counselling

Much research has identified that carers have high rates of anxiety and depression (e.g. Iconomou *et al.* 2001), and that psychosocial support should be provided in the form of therapeutic groups or opportunities for counselling. These interventions are based on the assumption that 'it is good to talk' and that in sharing experiences, carers have the opportunity to have their experiences acknowledged and validated by others in similar circumstances. They also provide a learning experience and an opportunity for emotional off-loading away from the cared for person. While these interventions may be useful for a few carers, generally it is found that they tend to attract very few people, and those that attend tend to be articulate middle class women. There are also practical problems in providing continuing care for the ill person while the carer is attending the support groups.

Respite

There are a number of models of respite provision in palliative care including planned and emergency care, provided by in-patient admissions, day care services and in home support such as 'night sitters' or intensive hospice-at-home schemes. These are based on the assumption that carers can be supported in their care giving role by being given a break (institutional respite admissions), having regular short breaks from caring (day care services) or having additional resources supplied in the home to provide intensive support (hospice-at-home services) or a good night's rest (night sitters). Despite respite facilities being widely available, a systematic review of respite in specialist palliative care found remarkably little research examining the effects of respite upon carer's welfare (Ingleton *et al.* 2003). The authors concluded that there was insufficient evidence to draw conclusions about the efficacy of offering respite care to support carers of patients with advanced disease.

Is caring for someone near the end of life the same as other types of caring?

In this final section, I will reflect on the special nature of caring of a person near the end of life, and the extent to which the carer's role is the same or different from any other type of caring. Thomas, Morris and Harman (2002) drew on a large study of carers for those with cancer to highlight the extent to which families share in the experience of illness. They differentiated between 'caring for' (care work tasks) and 'caring about' (emotional labour). The emphasis in the literature and in policy documents is on the 'caring for' elements in terms of counting the number of hours spent in direct care work and in enumerating physical tasks. This meant that at the early stages of cancer people did not recognize their companions as 'carers' because they were not engaged in physical care tasks. Thomas and Morris (2002) compared two alternative approaches to carers in the literature; the perspective taken by psychosocial oncology which tends to construe psychosocial needs of carers as indicative of psychological or psychiatric morbidity, and the sociological stance which emphasizes qualities of social life and social relationships. They argue that the psychosocial oncology perspective tends to see carers' needs as individual deficits and therefore suggests that interventions should focus on relieving the 'burden' of care by for example temporarily removing the cared for person such as in a respite admission or by providing psychological interventions such as counselling to promote personal coping skills in the carer. The alternative is to regard carers as embedded in complex patterns of social relationships from which they may draw both support and further problems.

Currently there is plenty of research evidence to indicate that carers have many challenges and demands but little evidence about how best to help them (Harding and Higginson 2003). There are a number of qualitative differences in carers providing end-of-life care compared to those providing continuing care to those with long-term chronic illness. Perhaps the most important factor is that there is no second chance to get things right once the person has died. Time together is very precious. Family carers may have made promises to their loved one, for example, to care for them at home, which may be very difficult to keep. Carers may feel under pressure to provide their loved one with a 'good death', however that is constructed. Moreover carers want to do their 'best' and get it 'right'. However, there are many 'scripts for dying' and there may be conflicts within families about what constitutes 'best' care, with some members wishing to pursue active treatment right to the end.

Care giving near the end-of-life may be highly emotional because of the impending sense of irrevocable loss. The nature of the terminal trajectory may influence the degree of exhaustion of the carer, for example, the dying phase may be characterized by a rapid and unpredictable decline compared to a slow protracted deterioration. There is timeliness in dying which is neither too fast or too slow but people do not normally have a choice over the speed of dying. Carers may experience considerable ambivalence about the anticipated loss, with on the one hand wishing to end the suffering of the ill person quickly, and on the other hand, not wanting to lose their loved one. They may oscillate between these conflicting desires, appearing contradictory to health care workers. Caring during a final illness is characterized by numerous losses, as the ill person withdraws from social life, becomes dependent and requires personal care (Evans 1994). These losses impact upon the family as social roles become renegotiated, for example a mother may no longer be able to provide physical care to her six-year-old son but can still help him to learn to read and write. When the dying period is very prolonged and the ill person becomes uncommunicative or has been sedated and is therefore unresponsive, the carer may start to experience anticipatory grief. This may involve some emotional withdrawal from the dying person.

The end-of-life period may be complicated by complex physical symptoms such as pain, breathlessness, fatigue, cachexia, cough, fungating, and discharging wounds which may make sustaining normal social relationships very difficult (Lawton 2000). Likewise, severe psychological distress such as depression may make the ill person very difficult to care for. It is therefore important that all symptoms are assessed and treated in line with the wishes of the patient and carer. However, intensive treatment may present challenges to the patient and family. Carers often want additional help but too many visits by health and social care workers may be perceived as invasive and too much of an intrusion into their home. For example, intensive home support such as hospice-at-home schemes, has been criticized by some people as medicalizing their home. Likewise, the admission of the ill person to a hospice or acute hospital may be perceived as helpful for the control of difficult symptoms or as a final betrayal, especially when the care delivered is perceived to be invasive or the environment is seen as too clinical. It is difficult for carers to achieve all they wish for the dying person, as many of the wishes may be contradictory—to keep their loved one with them as long as possible and to end their suffering. Health and social care workers can only strive to work alongside carers by acknowledging their essential contribution to the dying person and recognizing their own separate needs both before and after the death. Suggestions for supporting carers are provided in Box 3.

Box 3 Suggestions for Supporting Carers

- Recognizing their need to be treated with dignity and respect.
- Recognizing that they are not mere appendages of patients but have their own views, needs, and desires.
- Recognizing that carers have other social roles, responsibilities, and relationships.
- Recognizing that carers may not share the same worldviews, beliefs, attitudes, and culture as the patient.
- Recognizing that caring work involves more than physical tasks and that much caring activity is 'hidden'.
- Providing sufficient access to appropriate up-to-date information delivered in a style, language and at a pace that is compatible with the carer's wishes.
- Clear information about how to access additional information.
- Advice on how to access local and national carers support groups and facilities.
- Enabling them to make choices about becoming a carer, the extent of their caring activities and if and when they no longer wish to continue caring.

References

Barnard D, Towers A, Boston P, and Lambrinidou Y (2000) *Crossing Over: Narratives of Palliative Care.* Oxford University Press, Oxford.

Bowers BJ (1987) Inter-generational caregiving: adult caregivers and their ageing parents. *Advances in Nursing Science* **9**(2):20–31.

Crawford M, Rutter D, Manley C, *et al.* (2002) Systematic review of involving patients in the planning and development of health care. *British Medical Journal* **325**:1263–9.

Department of Health (1999/2000) *National Surveys of NHS Patients Cancer National Overview 1999/2000.* Department of Health, HMSO.

Dixon-Woods M (2001) Writing wrongs? An analysis of published discourses about the use of patient information leaflets. *Social Science and Medicine* **52**:1417–32.

Evans A (1994) Anticipatory grief: a theoretical challenge. *Palliative Medicine* **8**(2): 159–65.

Gott M, Stevens T, Small N, Ahmedzai SH (2002) User involvement in cancer care. *British Journal of Clinical Governance* **7**(2):81–5.

Greenberger H and Litwin H (2003) Can burdened caregivers be effective facilitators of elder care-recipient health care? *Journal of Advanced Nursing* **41**(4):332–41.

Harding R and Higginson IJ (2003) What is the best way to help caregivers in cancer and palliative care? A systematic literature review of interventions and their effectiveness. *Palliative Medicine* **17**:63–74.

Hawker R (1983) *The Interaction Between Nurses and Patients Relatives.* Unpublished PhD thesis, University of Exeter.

Hinton JM (1994*a*) Can home care maintain an acceptable quality of life for patients with terminal cancer and their relatives? *Palliative Medicine* **8**:183–96.

Hinton J (1994*b*) Which patients with terminal cancer are admitted from home care? *Palliative Medicine* **8**:197–210.

Iconomou G, Vagenakis AG, and Kalofonos HP (2001) The informational needs, satisfaction with communication, and psychological status of primary caregivers of cancer patients receiving chemotherapy. *Supportive Care in Cancer* **9**:591–6.

Ingleton C, Payne S, Nolan M, and Carey I (2003) Respite in palliative care: a review and discussion of the literature. *Palliative Medicine* **17**:567–75.

Lawton J (2000) *The Dying Process. Patients' Experiences of Palliative Care.* Routledge, London.

Low JTS, Payne S, and Roderick P (1999) The impact of stroke on informal carers: a literature review. *Social Science and Medicine* **49**(6):711–25.

Maher J and Green H (2002) *Carers 2000 Office of National Statistics.* The Stationery Office, London.

Neufeld A and Harrison MJ (2003) Unfulfilled expectations and negative interactions: non-support in the relationships of women caregivers. *Journal of Advanced Nursing* **41**(4):323–31.

Nolan M (2001) Positive aspects of caring. In Payne S and Ellis-Hill C (ed.) *Chronic and Terminal Illness: New Perspectives in Caring and Carers.* Oxford University Press, Oxford.

Nolan M, Grant G, and Keady J (1995) Developing a typology of family care: implications for nurses and other service providers. *Journal of Advanced Nursing* **21**:256–65.

Nolan M, Grant G, and Keady J (1996) The carer's act: realising the potential. *British Journal of Community Health Nursing* **1**(6):317–22.

Payne S and Ellis-Hill C (ed.) (2001) *Chronic and Terminal Illness: New Perspectives in Caring and Carers.* Oxford University Press, Oxford.

Rook KS and Pietromonaco P (1987) Close relationships: ties that heal or ties that bind? In Jones WH and Perlman D (ed.) *Advances in Personal Relationships: A Research Annual.* JAI Press, Greenwich.

Segal J and Simkins J (1993) *My Mum Needs Me: Helping Children with Ill or Disabled Parents.* Penguin Books, London.

Seymour JE, Clark D, Gott M, Bellamy G, and Ahmedzai S (2002) Good deaths, bad deaths: older people's assessments of risks and benefits in the use of morphine and terminal sedation in end of life care. *Health, Risk and Society* **4**(3):287–304.

Small N and Rhodes P (2000) *Too Ill to Talk? User Involvement in Palliative Care.* Routledge, London.

Smith P (2001) Who is a carer? Experiences of family caregivers in palliative care. In Payne S and Ellis-Hill C (ed.) *Chronic and Terminal Illness: New Perspectives in Caring and Carers.* Oxford University Press, Oxford.

The National Cancer Alliance (1996) *"Patient-Centred Cancer Services"? What Patients Say.* The National Cancer Alliance, Oxford.

The A-M (2002) *Palliative Care and Communication: Experiences in the Clinic.* Open University Press, Buckingham.

Thomas C, Morris SM, and Harman JC (2002) Companions through cancer: the care given by informal carers in cancer contexts. *Social Science and Medicine* **54**(4):529–44.

Thomas C and Morris SM (2002) Informal carers in cancer contexts. *European Journal of Cancer Care* **11**:178–82.

Twigg J and Atkin K (1994) *Carers Perceived.* Open University Press, Buckingham.

Walker A (1996) *Young Carers and their Families.* HMSO, London.

Index